Gender and Groupwork

Thinking about gender can enrich the work of all groupwork practitioners and can make a real difference in people's lives. Based on practice experience in both the UK and the USA, *Gender and Groupwork* brings together the best of groupwork knowledge, skills and values in a true transatlantic partnership.

The book summarises the history of gender-based groups for both women and men and outlines a wide range of exciting and challenging examples of groups in different contexts. Often moving, and always engrossing, these accounts encompass groups for older women, for women with learning difficulties, for minority ethnic women and women facing inequalities in health care. Innovative work with homeless people, with caregivers and lesbian and gay youth is described in detail, and there is a particular focus on domestic violence, where groups can often be the intervention of choice.

Gender and Groupwork demonstrates that, despite the challenges of post-structuralism and postmodernism, the practice of groupwork is alive and well. It provides new ideas and new models to help move practice forward, making it a welcome addition to the groupwork literature.

Marcia B. Cohen is Professor of Social Work at the University of New England, USA. **Audrey Mullender** is Professor of Social Work at the University of Warwick, UK.

Gender and Groupwork

Edited by Marcia B. Cohen and
Audrey Mullender

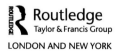 Routledge
Taylor & Francis Group

LONDON AND NEW YORK

First published 2003
by Routledge
2 Park Square, Milton Park, Abingdon, Oxfordshire OX14 4RN

Simultaneously published in the USA and Canada
by Routledge
711 Third Avenue, New York, NY 10017

Routledge is an imprint of the Taylor & Francis Group

Selection and editorial matter © 2003 Marcia B. Cohen and Audrey Mullender;
© individual chapters the contributors

Typeset in Times New Roman by
Keystroke, Jacaranda Lodge, Wolverhampton

British Library Cataloguing in Publication Data
A catalogue record for this book is available from the British Library

Library of Congress Cataloging in Publication Data
A catalog record for this book has been requested

ISBN 0–415–08057–6 (pbk)
ISBN 0–415–08056–8 (hbk)

Dedication

To David and John, with love, and in memory of Roísín

Contents

Acknowledgements

We would like to offer our sincere thanks to the following: all our contributors, without whose hard work this book would not have been possible, Edwina Welham, Michelle Bacca, Sonia Pati and Victoria Gibbins at Routledge for their kind assistance at all stages of this project, Ann Macfarlane MBE for her advice on disability issues, Dr Cathy Humphreys for expertise on postmodernism, Sylvia Moore for her help in preparing the manuscript, and each other for first-rate transatlantic collaboration and for always worrying about different things at different times so the other was free to problem-solve. We also celebrate the groupworkers and group members whose work is reflected throughout this book. In time-honoured fashion, we have benefited enormously from the input and support of all the forementioned, but the responsibility for any errors or infelicities remains with us.

Chapter 1

Introduction

Audrey Mullender and Marcia B. Cohen

This book has had a long gestation. The idea for it first arose ten years ago when women's groups were plentiful and both groupwork and feminist practice were at the core of the social work curriculum. It seemed natural, then, to conceive of a book that would help groupworkers develop awareness and skill in handling the gender issues in their practice, and that would, at the same time, strengthen in the literature on gender a particularly important way of working with women to change their lives. It was to have been a single-authored work but, for various reasons (chiefly competing research priorities), that book did not get written and the idea was laid to rest. Only when we discovered how fruitful our collaboration could be (Cohen and Mullender 2000), and explored our shared interests in women's issues, as well as in groups, was the project reborn – this time as one we decided to undertake together as editors of a collection that would explore whether 'gender and groupwork' still has meaning in the twenty-first century.

Immediately, a new set of challenges was created. A transatlantic co-operation would mean writing for two different audiences, and this has meant persuading the publisher to allow this book to be 'bi-lingual', by which we mean that it alternates between UK and US use of English (spelling, punctuation, grammar and expression – reviewers please note that variant styles are not uncorrected errors!). Most centrally, even 'groupwork' (UK) or 'group work' (USA) is written in two different ways throughout the book, depending on the provenance of any particular chapter. We have compromised on UK style for the introductory and concluding chapters, in recognition of our London-based publishing house. But, of course, the two nations that straddle the Atlantic are divided by more than a common language (to paraphrase the aphorism attributed to Winston Churchill and echoing similar thoughts of Oscar Wilde, George Bernard Shaw, Bertrand Russell and Dylan Thomas in the UK and Mark Twain in the USA). Groups have developed their own body of literature and practice wisdom in the two countries, although it has been interesting to note the transferability of practice skills and values (and similarly with the excellent Canadian and Australian contributions to this volume). Contributors have written from their own experiences and perspectives, in their own national context. The concluding chapter will attempt to pull together our ideas about where this leaves us.

Most apparent to us as editors was a difference in theoretical outlook between the social sciences more generally in the two countries. Britain has been in the direct line of an outpouring of postmodernist and poststructuralist ideas from France that has affected social work theory rather less substantially in the USA, though educators there are familiar with the body of ideas. In the UK, it has been scarcely possible for several years now to talk about any collective action for change without encountering strident accusations of essentialism, modernism or universalism (i.e. the view that seeking change at the societal level oversimplifies the degree of commonality between people and their goals, the nature of power, and the extent to which human beings move towards progress), while the term 'empowerment' has become a positive embarrassment, again in the face of Foucauldian reflections that power is far more fragmented than Marxist or feminist meta-narratives or other 'grand theories' would suggest. British social work writing has had to encompass both an awareness of difference and diversity (which arguably is not as new as is made out – a point to which we shall return below and in the concluding chapter) and the rise of subjectivity and relativism to a point at which there seemed little potential for shared awareness in groups, let alone any common goals for change. In the USA, in contrast, empowerment practice continues to be explored, examined and expanded upon. The toll taken by Thatcherite and Reaganite 'me-first' politics and the advent of managerialist regulation within social work agencies under a succession of administrations in both countries have similarly made groupwork appear old-hat. Certainly, there has been a rapid decline in the UK in practising, teaching and writing about groupwork as a method. As Ward (1998: 149) states, '"groupwork" seems . . . to have faded from view'. In the USA, while groups themselves are quite prevalent in agency settings, there are fewer and fewer groupworkers trained to facilitate them. At the same time, the backlash against feminism (Faludi 1992) and against anti-oppressive practice (Dominelli 1998), together with the postmodernist–poststructuralist trend against single-issue groups and towards fragmentation of identities, have added to the decline in women's groups and in practitioners' willingness to profess themselves feminists (White 1995).

Given this diluting of their medium, how aware are groupworkers these days of gender issues in their practice? Does (and should) gender awareness affect the way they work – for example, do men and women, girls and boys, have different needs in groups? And what about the diversity within those categories – is it so extreme that 'gender' is no longer a useful organizing idea? Has groupwork theory – ideas about dynamics, roles, stages and other aspects of the process in groups – kept pace with this more complex thinking about gender or are we still trying to impose outmoded notions on people who have moved on in the ways they conceive of their lives? What effect does all this have on the practice?

Also, just as we can ask whether there is gender in groups, is there groupwork in gender studies? For example, how aware are feminists (and other writers about women), or those involved in developing theories of masculinity, of the history of groupwork in drawing out the key issues in men's and women's lives? Are agendas of change still relevant, or is gender studies now purely an intellectual arena, far removed from the applied disciplines like social work?

When we bring the two areas together – gender and groupwork – are there fully fledged models that have attempted to make this conjunction? Notably, what is (or was) 'feminist groupwork'? What principles does it reflect and how does it relate to empowerment groupwork, social action groupwork, and other approaches that aim to help group members identify and build on their strengths? How has any of these stood up in the face of postmodernist and poststructuralist challenges to essentialist and dichotomized thinking about the categories 'male' and 'female' and to 'top–down' ideas of power? These are some of the questions we will engage with in this book, through discussion and examples from practice.

The background – in the UK

Looking back over the UK literature on groupwork, there has been little systematic analysis of gender as a factor in the development of groupwork theory. It is true that anti-sexism and provision for women in groups became increasingly present as an issue (contrast Brown's third edition in 1992 with the two earlier editions), largely as a result of wider concerns, first with anti-discriminatory or anti-oppressive practice (e.g. Mullender and Ward 1991) and then with the diversity agenda within postmodernism (e.g. Doel and Sawdon 1999). Hence gender has been there as part of the fabric of groupwork, and has often been a consideration in group task or content, but with little rigorous disentangling of what this means in a technical or analytical sense.

In the journal *Groupwork*, a good number of accounts of women's groups have appeared over the years, and a few of groups for men. One early overview of the literature on women's groups (Fitzgerald 1989) consisted of a set of abstracts and attempted little in the way of a conceptual framework. Following that, there appeared many accounts of particular groups that happened to be single-sex, rather than papers about gender in groups as such. They dealt with substantive content on the experiences of refugee women (Tribe and Shackman 1989), sexually abused girls (Craig 1990), mothers of sexually abused children (Masson and Erooga 1990; Dobbin and Evans 1994; Otway and Peake 1994), teenage pregnancy (Norman 1994), depression (Trevithick 1995) and eating disorders (Ball and Norman 1996), for example. There were also one or two groups for women workers themselves, as managers (Fawcett 1994) and as mental health providers (Holstein and Laperdon-Addison 1994), both of these appearing in the special issue 'Groupwork with Women', edited by Claire Wintram in 1994, which also contained several of the user group examples. Women offenders were seen as offenders with women's problems (Mistry 1989; Barnett *et al*. 1990; Jones *et al*. 1991) and as offending in different ways from men and for different reasons. Groups for men were also in evidence (Cowburn 1990; Erooga *et al*. 1990; Bensted *et al*. 1994; Mullender 1996) – chiefly as perpetrators of sexual abuse, domestic violence and crime more generally – as were groups for boys (Craig 1988; Clarke and Aimable 1990; Dixon and Phillips 1994), often as survivors of child sexual abuse. Most practitioners used the group to deal with gendered themes or gendered aspects of wider issues, and most of the accounts do draw out some general points about feminist process in groupwork. However, few authors offered much comment on the detail of that process, and it is not apparent that many had, in fact, re-thought, or strayed far from, conventional groupwork theory.

In social work practice more broadly, feminist authors accorded groupwork a special place, as offering women an effective way of obtaining support (Dominelli and McLeod 1989). It was also seen as enabling social workers themselves to offer and receive mutual support (Hanmer and Statham 1988). There were hidden riches of groupwork accounts, including groups for black women, lesbian and working-class women, in self-help manuals, particularly from the mental health sector. The Women's Therapy Centre (see Ernst and Goodison 1981; Krzowski and Land 1988) and Women in MIND (1986), for example, which had a grounding in psychoanalytic approaches, emphasized groups, drop-ins, networks, community education classes and support projects as important opportunities for women to sustain or regain their mental and emotional health. Students running feminist groups used them as the subject of their Master's dissertations (Evans 1985; Donnelly 1986), and this included a focus on feminist groupwork in the statutory sector, notably in relation to child care concerns where women tended to be labelled in casework contexts as inadequate mothers.

Overall, there was no single method for working with women. The full range of groupwork methods was in evidence, including task-centred activities (Clarke and Aimable 1990), art therapy (Otway 1993), social action (Butler 1994) and psychotherapy (Trevithick 1995). Most of the groupwork technique in use was 'unisex', and was largely unquestioned. If there was a 'feminist groupwork', we see it most clearly in the paper by Mistry (1989) and particularly in the book-length account by Butler and Wintram (1991), all of whom were writing about groups they themselves had run. The method used by Butler and Wintram, in what is certainly the most extended contribution to the UK literature on gender and groupwork, was broadly that of consciousness-raising. Interestingly, they were already conveying a strong sense of the diversity within the category of 'woman', as early as 1991. We return to this below.

The background – in the USA

In contrast to the UK, there have been a number of analyses of gender and of groupwork in the USA. In addition to accounts of particular groups of men and women (including Knight 1990; Lovell *et al.* 1992; Pence 1993; Reid *et al.* 1995; Russell 1995; Brannen and Rubin 1996; Sharf 1997; Miller *et al.* 2000) that parallel those in the UK literature described above, there is a body of literature concerned explicitly with gender in groups, which has directly influenced our understanding of group dynamics and processes.

Reed and Garvin were among the earliest contributors to this literature, and they have remained active in this area of enquiry. Much of their work has focused on generating an in-depth view of gender within the context of feminist groupwork principles. A *Social Work With Groups* special issue in 1983, which they edited, marked the first major contribution to the exploration of gender in the US groupwork literature. The editors' own overview article, which served as an introduction, directly addressed the dimension of gender in social groupwork, arguing that issues of gender should be of central importance to groupworkers. Reed and Garvin set the stage for further analysis in their identification of key concepts in understanding gender stereotyping and status differences as they relate to work with groups, and highlighted the problem of gender bias in practice. They also pointed to the paucity of gender considerations in practice theory and research, inviting other gender-conscious groupworkers to help fill the identified gaps in practice knowledge, particularly in strengthening our understanding of the interaction between the gender, ethnicity and age of group leaders and members, the overlaps between mental illness and gender issues, the relationship between sexual orientation and gender identity in the context of groupwork, and the need to develop a gendered analysis of all practice models and approaches used by groupworkers.

Other articles in that 1983 issue of *Social Work With Groups* provide a glimpse of the flowering of gender-based groupwork at that time. They included a discussion of a group of male professionals focused on an exploration of male gender roles as they impacted on members' responsiveness to feminist concerns (Kaufman and Timmers 1983), an examination of the gender bias in social skills' training groups (Gambrill and Richey 1983), a discussion of a group which actively explored gender issues in domestic violence situations (Currie *et al.* 1983) an analysis of the intersection of sexual orientation and gender role stereotyping (Morson and McInnis 1983) and an evaluation of the impact of gender roles and attitudes in the context of a women's consciousness-raising group for psychiatrically labelled women (Adolph 1983). This special issue of *Social Work With Groups* was groundbreaking in its multifaceted and gendered exploration of groupwork. It was followed, although not for several years, by further scholarship that addressed Garvin and Reed's call for research and theory to place the issue of gender centre-stage in the arena of group practice.

One noteworthy example was Van Nostrand's book *Gender-Responsible Leadership* (1993), which provided a very thorough analysis of subtle and not so subtle gender bias in the leadership of a wide variety of mixed-gender groups. Gender bias is understood as reflecting the sexism prevalent in our society, which, if allowed to go unexamined, serves to reinforce it. Using research findings and group examples to underscore her argument, Van Nostrand provided a very detailed discussion of the power of group facilitators, either to collude with or combat manifestations of male entitlement. This remains a highly practical sourcebook for group leadership, actively promoting gender equity through an awareness of the interconnectedness of patriarchy, power, group process and leadership. The author gives concrete examples of the leader's role in: detecting gender biases; being aware of any tendencies towards gender-oriented favouritism; the power of language in reinforcing male privilege; the potential for rigid gender roles to impede growth; the impact of different leadership styles; and a series of interventions aimed at encouraging gender equity within a group.

A number of research studies were conducted in the USA in the 1990s, focused on the impact of gender on group leadership (Shimanoff and Jenkins 1991; Eagly *et al.* 1992; Kent and Moss 1994; Cooper 1997; Kolb 1997). These discussions lack Van Nostrand's socio-political analysis and do not include specific applications for group leaders, but they are useful in bolstering the body of data that points to the significance of gender in group leadership.

Garvin and Reed have themselves continued to make significant contributions to the literature on gender and groups (1994, 1995), applying core feminist principles to social groupwork and scrutinizing the gendering process in groups. They carefully draw the interconnections between feminist theory and groupwork: historical, epistemological and ideological. Pointing out that many features of modern feminist practice were developed in group settings, they underscore the shared historical roots of feminism and social groupwork. They apply a feminist critique of the social goals, remedial, reciprocal and task-group models of social groupwork, and contrast those practice approaches with a feminist groupwork. The model developed by Garvin and Reed incorporates the personal, interpersonal and social action goals of the other four models while emphasizing the identification of gender issues and the rectification of power imbalance based on gender. The various social and psychological theories of change encompassed by earlier models are reconstructed here in the light of contemporary feminist theory. The implications of this feminist groupwork model for the role of the worker and the group member are carefully delineated, with an emphasis on eliminating hierarchy within the group, engaging in sex-role analysis, examining gendering practices, exploring the connections between the personal and the political, and striving for a non-oppressive society. This coupling of theory and practice, joining feminism and groupwork, provides clear principles for feminist groupwork practitioners.

Saulnier's recent (2000) scholarship expands on the analysis of feminist theory and groupwork. Her in-depth review of five different branches of feminist theory provides a careful delineation of some of the frameworks that inform feminist groupwork. Drawing on her research with groups of women, Saulnier articulates the goals and processes that distinguish groupwork applications of liberal feminism, cultural feminism, postmodern feminism, womanism and radical feminism. Using a framework that teases out theoretical goals, group focus, group process and group goals, she brings clarity to the relevance of feminist theory to social groupwork while distinguishing between different bodies of feminist thought.

This framework portrays, first, liberal feminism as having the goal of gaining equal access to existing services, rights and privacy, rather than seeking new or different rights or resources. Groups informed by liberal feminism tend to focus on such topics as problem drinking and dysfunctional familial relationships. Using processes including twelve-step programmes (used by Alcoholics Anonymous), counselling and psycho-education, liberal feminist groups seek to help members increase their self-esteem and assertiveness while gaining skills and a sense of self-competence.

Second, cultural feminism, in Saulnier's framework, is characterized by goals revolving around the restructuring of society through the development of women's culture, values and spirituality. Cultural feminist groups have a broad range of topical foci, many evolving from twelve-step or other recovery programmes. The processes most frequently used in these groups are consciousness-raising, self-help and support. Cultural feminist groups embrace goals of political analysis, celebrating womanhood, and creating new religious and spiritual experiences for women.

Third, postmodern feminism, in contrast, has the goals of articulating a feminist viewpoint, analysing the impact of the social world on women, and examining power and knowledge for the purpose of societal transformation. Groups informed by postmodernist feminism have tended to be popular among upper-middle-class women, lesbians in particular, who have sought as their primary group focus networking and creating connections. The most frequently used processes in postmodern feminist groups are, as Saulnier describes them, bibliotherapy, education and support. These groups have as their goals: networking, building community support and changing how people talk and think about feminism.

Fourth, womanist feminism focuses on the intersection of gender and race within society. Its goals are activist in nature, clustering around social action and social change, articulating ethnic consciousness and actively resisting multiple systems of oppression. The focus of womanist groups reflects their composition, lesbians and women of colour being central topics as well as group participants. Processes used in womanist groups are self-empowerment, community building, racial consciousness-raising and forced recognition, by societal power structures, of communities of colour.

Finally, radical feminism, as distinguished in Saulnier's outline, incorporates the goals of making connections between the personal and the political, eliminating male privilege, healing internalized sexism, protecting women from male violence, and the restructuring of society. The group approach most associated with this perspective is the 'empowerment institute', utilizing group processes such as consciousness-raising, support, skill development and the production of action plans. The objectives of radical feminist groups include healing the injuries wrought by patriarchy, challenging patriarchal indoctrination and empowering women to take action for social change.

Saulnier suggests that despite the differences among the branches of feminist theory informing these different types of groups, there are common themes of support, consciousness-raising and empowerment, and of moving from personal to political concerns, which characterize most feminist groupwork. Effective feminist group facilitation necessitates that workers be aware of the similarities and differences between these theoretical perspectives and sensitive to their implications for groupwork practice.

The US groupwork literature has also included explorations of gender and race within a groupwork context (Hirayama and Hirayama 1985; Gutiérrez 1990; Davis *et al.* 1996; Raja 1998; Gutiérrez and Lewis 1999). The recent work of Gutiérrez and Lewis (1999) has been instrumental in increasing our understanding of the intersection of gender and race in groups. As Chapter 11 of this volume explains, Lewis and Gutiérrez highlight the interactional nature of ethnicity and gender in empowerment-oriented work with groups. Multicultural empowering group practitioners are characterized as having a heightened sensitivity to the impact on group process of skin colour, ethnicity, sexual orientation, social class and gender. Emphasizing the use of empowerment techniques, Gutiérrez and Lewis (1999) identify a series of issues to be addressed in groups of women of colour: identifying and eliminating the unconscious use of stereotypes; attending to issues of power; and addressing issues of oppression and gender construction based on bicultural and multicultural socialization. A recurrent theme in their work is the critical importance of openly engaging with issues of similarity and difference within groups, particularly with regard to gender and ethnicity.

Sensitivity to racism and sexism, a heightened awareness of and willingness to address gender and racial stereotyping, and the celebration of diversity are emphasized in much of the US literature on gender, ethnicity and groupwork (Hirayama and Hirayama 1985; Gutiérrez 1990; Raja 1998). These authors all note the strong contribution of feminist theory to groupwork in this domain, particularly its emphasis on the impact of the societal context, its awareness of power dynamics and its strong orientation to empowerment.

Research and writing from the Stone Center at Wellesley College (Jordan *et al.* 1991) marks a turning point in the development of gender-conscious theory for practice. Self-in-relation provides a clearly articulated, gender-sensitive practice theory that has been applied to psychodynamic group therapy by DeChant (1996) and to a much broader spectrum of treatment- and task-oriented groups by Schiller (1995, 1997). The concepts of mutuality, empathy, connection and relationship are central to self-in-relation theory. As Schiller describes in Chapter 2 of this volume, the integration of self-in-relation theory with classical group development models generates a very different perspective on how groups can develop and grow over time. Schiller's landmark work on the relational model of group development portrays a pathway taken by many women's groups, and even some mixed-gender groups, in which conflict does not emerge until late in group development when mutuality and connection are present, and then takes the form of constructive challenge rather than a vying for power and control. The relational model has profoundly influenced our understanding of the impact of gender on groupwork, particularly with regard to the nature and timing of connection, mutuality, empathy, challenge and conflict.

Themes that emerge from the US literature on gender and groupwork, overall, include creating support networks, mutuality and connection, consciousness-raising, moving from the personal to the political, awareness of social context and empower-ment. All of these will recur throughout this book, albeit in forms that are now perhaps more aware of difference and diversity, overlaps and interconnections between a range of oppressions, and less willing to regard 'women' as a homogeneous category. This has occurred in response to a postmodernist agenda which we will now explore.

Empowerment and postmodernism

Feminism and groupwork have always found a natural home together in empowerment agendas, and this has made them sitting targets for postmodernist charges of essentialism (see Thompson 1998 for an explanation in an anti-discriminatory social work context). There are two aspects to this challenge: first, the need to see diversity and multiple subjectivities within any social grouping; and, second, the need for a more contemporary analysis of power that does not see it purely as 'top down' in a simplistic notion of oppression but allows for individual agency and resistance from the 'bottom up'. At the same time, it is important to avoid the assumption that coming together or organizing together in groups is no longer necessary, helpful or possible.

We have moved beyond one feminism to many, and this means that group-workers must now ask when proposing any new group: 'which women benefit, how much, at what costs, compared to which alternatives[?]' (Rhode 1989: 317, quoted in Figueira-McDonough 1998: 19). We cannot assume that any particular woman's group is automatically good for all its members. It is crucial to work hard to ensure that no individual woman feels excluded from a group because she is subjectively not only female but also black or of dual heritage, lesbian, poor, disabled or older. (This list could, of course, be considerably longer.) On the other hand, this approach could lead to excessive fragmentation. We cannot base practice on an individualism that denies social interconnectedness, any more than we can allow enforced collectivization or outmodedly modernist assumptions of universal justice to deny individual difference or diversity. We have to see the group around the individual as much as the individual within the group.

A number of authors in recent years have attempted to move us beyond the initially paralysing self-questioning induced by the postcolonialist, postmodernist and poststructuralist challenges to any form of collective identity or action. While Leonard (1997; British, based in Canada) has undoubtedly led the way for social work in beginning to move out of the conceptual impasse into an 'emancipatory project' for social welfare, theorists in Australia (Pease and Fook 1999; Healy 2000) and the UK (Batsleer and Humphries 2000) have extended this thinking into detailed possibilities for 'critical', 'progressive' or 'transformative' practice. Others are also meeting the postmodernist challenge head-on by using it as the basis of new practice methods such as the narrative approach developed by Michael White at the Dulwich Centre in Adelaide, Australia (see, for example, White 1988–89 and 1991) and constructive social work in the UK (Parton and O'Byrne 2000). Though developed primarily as one-to-one methods, these can certainly be used in groups. Alternative mental health projects in Australia, for example (Community Mental Health Project 1997), have taken as a starting point the idea that knowledge is historically and culturally specific and that we must listen to the voices of individuals previously silenced by dominant discourses if we are to understand and work with them, for example through helping them tell the story of their lives in a different way so that they feel more worthy and less de-skilled. There is room within the new story to name injustice and to explore relations of power, though workers and project users are themselves seen as verbally deconstructing and dismantling existing power relations in ways that some might see as under-estimating the self-seeking of interest groups in the wider society in maintaining distancing and 'othering' mechanisms. At least collective awareness once more feels a possibility in a way that puts groups back on the agenda, albeit far more constrained in their ambitions. We are no longer setting out to change the world, but we can still engage with important processes of challenge and development at other levels.

To what extent is this something new? Is it just empowerment wearing a fresh suit of clothes? Certainly, we consider any assumption that earlier work on women's empowerment through groups was always essentialist to be oversimplified and unfair. On close examination, the diversity agenda has been there in the groupwork literature for at least the last decade. This was particularly so in relation to ethnicity (Rhule 1988; Mistry and Brown 1991, 1997; Muir and Notta 1993; Francis-Spence 1994) – though this was largely about black women, with Mistry and Brown (1997) noting that black men's groups were a striking omission – and socio-economic status (Bodinham and Weinstein 1991; Otway 1993; Butler 1994; Wintram *et al.* 1994) often overlapping with service-user status around lone motherhood and child care concerns. Hearing the stories of socially excluded individuals and groups is central to empowerment. The chief empowerment model in UK groupwork, Mullender and Ward's 'self-directed groupwork' (1991), was based on principles of recognizing skills and abilities in all individuals, hearing silenced voices, and working jointly and reflexively with service users in ways that did not privilege professional knowledge. Nor did it assume top–down power as the only influence. Rather, individual agency and resistance were key to the campaigning and activism undertaken. The understanding of gender was not essentialist, making specific mention of Asian women, younger and older women, class boundaries, and so on (see also Butler and Wintram 1991). There is at least some sense in which it is the language rather than the underlying aims that has altered. It is important though, in our underpinning understanding, to avoid making claims to provide explanations for all women's social experiences or assumptions of dichotomy between all women and all men. Equally, in our practice, it is vital always to question who is motivating and steering change and for whose benefit (bottom up as well as top down), and who is being included in or excluded from any group. There remains a role for feminism in bringing forward these new understandings (Williams 1996; Fawcett *et al.* 2000; Dominelli forthcoming), provided that it is a feminism of global diversity and critical awareness.

Because social science theory has moved on so fast, while groupwork has been in something of a decline, there is an unevenness of awareness in the chapters that follow. Some are more informed by groupwork theory and less aware of diversity and social agency, while in others the opposite applies. A few encompass both theoretical fields. All bring an in-depth knowledge of their particular topics, and none will be wholly familiar to the entire readership of this book since they have flourished in different parts of the world. Drawn together in this volume, they suggest that concerns with gender in groups remain alive and well and that single-sex and mixed groups for men, women and children can all gain from a more gendered awareness on the part both of the group leaders and of the members.

Conclusion

Taken as a whole, this book engages with gender at a level of complexity that covers myriad experiences within the categories 'male' and 'female' and does not see these as polarized – notably in the chapter by DeLois in which one group member is shown to move between these categorizations. The key questions in all this have to remain, though, whether women and girls can gain from being in single-sex groups something that is otherwise not available to them, whether groups can challenge abusive men to change their behaviour and attitudes towards women, and whether mixed-sex groups can meet the needs of both women and men, girls and boys, rather than those of one sex at the expense of the other. The challenge is to offer these strengths of groupwork without the denial of some people's experience that was inherent in essentialist or universalist understandings of gender and patriarchy.

In the chapters that follow, issues of gender and groupwork are explored in relation to women and men as diverse social groupings, including: profeminist men, abusive men, abused women, child witnesses of woman abuse, sexual minorities, disabled people, minority ethnic women, older women, homeless women, caregivers and those experiencing oppression due to gender and health care inequalities. This broad array of topics emphasizes the commonalities and diversity within 'gender', as well as the interaction between various forms of oppression, marginalization or exclusion. The practice issues inherent in the facilitation, dynamics, process and stages of groups are explored from a multilayered gender perspective. We begin with Schiller's more analytical chapter, illustrating the extent to which a gendered framework can challenge received wisdom in groupwork theory and raising themes that will recur throughout the book, before moving into historical overviews of women's and men's experiences in feminist and profeminist groups, and then into more detailed practice-related examples.

References

Adolf, M. (1983) 'The all-women's consciousness raising group as a component for treatment of mental illness', *Social Work With Groups*, 6, 3–4: 117–31.
Ball, J. and Norman, A. (1996) '"Without the group I'd still be eating half the Co-op": an example of groupwork with women who use food', *Groupwork*, 9, 1: 48–61.
Barnett, S., Corder, F. and Jehu, D. (1990) 'Group treatment for women sex offenders against children', *Groupwork*, 3, 2: 191–203.

Batsleer, J. and Humphries, B. (eds) (2000) *Welfare, Exclusion and Political Agency*, London: Routledge.

Bensted, J., Brown, A., Forbes, C. and Wall, R. (1994) 'Men working with men in groups: masculinity and crime', *Groupwork*, 7, 1: 37–49.

Bodinham, H. and Weinstein, J. (1991) 'Making authority accountable: the experience of a statutory based women's group', *Groupwork*, 4, 1: 22–30.

Brannen, S. and Rubin, A. (1996) 'Comparing the effectiveness of gender specific and couples groups in a court-mandated spouse abuse treatment program', *Research on Social Work Practice*, 6, 4: 405–24.

Brown, A. (1992) *Groupwork*, 3rd edition, Aldershot: Ashgate.

Butler, S. (1994) '"All I've got in my purse is mothballs!" The social action women's group', *Groupwork*, 7, 2: 163–79.

Butler, S. and Wintram, C. (1991) *Feminist Groupwork*, London: Sage.

Clarke, P. and Aimable, A. (1990) 'Groupwork techniques in a residential primary school for emotionally disturbed boys', *Groupwork*, 3, 1: 36–48.

Cohen, M.B. and Mullender, A. (2000) 'The personal in the political: exploring the group work continuum from individual to social change goals', *Social Work With Groups*, 22, 1: 13–31.

Community Mental Health Project (1997) 'Companions on a journey: an exploration of an alternative community mental health project', *Dulwich Centre Newsletter*, no. 1 of 1997: 6–16. (Published in Adelaide, Australia.)

Cooper, V. (1997) 'Homophilly or the Queen Bee Syndrome: female evaluation of female leadership', *Small Group Research*, 28, 4: 483–500.

Cowburn, M. (1990) 'Work with male sex offenders in groups', *Groupwork*, 3, 2: 157–71.

Craig, E. (1990) 'Starting the journey: enhancing the therapeutic elements of groupwork for adolescent female child sexual abuse victims', *Groupwork*, 3, 2: 103–17.

Craig, R. (1988) 'Structured activities with adolescent boys', *Groupwork*, 1, 1: 48–59.

Currie, D.W., Buckley, L.B., Miller, D. and Rolfe, T.A. (1983) 'Treatment groups for violent men: two approaches', *Social Work With Groups* 6, 3–4: 177–95.

Davis, L.E., Cheng, L.C., and Strube, M.J. (1996) 'Differential effects of racial composition on male and female groups: implications for group work practice', *Social Work Research*, 20, 3: 157–66.

DeChant, B. (ed.) (1996) *Women and Group Psychotherapy: Theory and Practice*, New York: Guilford Press.

Dixon, G. and Phillips, M. (1994) 'A psychotherapeutic group for boys who have been sexually abused', *Groupwork*, 7, 1: 79–95.

Dobbin, D. and Evans, S. (1994) 'Staying alive in difficult times: the experience of groupwork with mothers of children who have been sexually abused', *Groupwork*, 7, 2: 117–24.

Doel, M. and Sawdon, C. (1999) *The Essential Groupworker: Teaching and Learning Creative Groupwork*, London: Jessica Kingsley.

Dominelli, L. (1998) 'Anti-oppressive practice in context', in R. Adams, L. Dominelli and M. Payne (eds) *Social Work: Themes, Issues and Critical Debates*, Basingstoke: Macmillan.

Dominelli, L. (2002) *Feminist Social Work Theory and Practice*, Basingstoke: Palgrave.

Dominelli, L. and McLeod, E. (1989) *Feminist Social Work*, Basingstoke: Macmillan.

Donnelly, A. (1986) *Feminist Social Work with a Women's Group*, Social Work Monograph 41, Norwich: University of East Anglia.

Eagly, A.H., Makhijani, M.G., and Klonsky, B.G. (1992) 'Gender and evaluation of leaders: a meta-analysis', *Psychological Bulletin*, 111: 3–22.

Ernst, S. and Goodison, L. (1981) *In Our Own Hands: A Book of Self-Help Therapy*, London: The Women's Press.

Erooga, M., Clark, P. and Bentley, M. (1990) 'Protection, control, treatment: groupwork with child sexual abuse', *Groupwork*, 3, 2: 172–90.

Evans, D. (1985) 'Developing feminist groups in statutory practice: a case study of a women's group in "Smalltown"', unpublished MA/CQSW dissertation, Coventry: University of Warwick, Department of Applied Social Studies (cited in Dominelli and McLeod 1989).

Faludi, S. (1992) *Backlash: The Undeclared War Against Women*, London: Vintage.

Fawcett, J. (1994) 'Promoting positive images: the role of groupwork in promoting women managers within organisations', *Groupwork*, 7, 2: 145–52.

Fawcett, B., Featherstone, B., Fook, J. and Rossiter, A. (2000) *Practice and Research in Social Work: Postmodern Feminist Perspectives*, London: Routledge.

Figueira-McDonough, J. (1998) 'Toward a gender-integrated knowledge in social work', in Figueira-McDonough, J., Netting, F.E. and Nichols-Casebolt, A. (eds) *The Role of Gender in Practice Knowledge: Claiming Half the Human Experience*, New York and London: Garland Publishing.

Fitzgerald, C. (1989) 'Searching the literature on women's groups', *Groupwork*, 2, 2: 167–73.

Francis-Spence, M. (1994) 'Groupwork and black women: viewing networks as groups', *Groupwork*, 7, 2: 109–16.

Gambrill, E. and Richey, C.A. (1983) 'Gender issues related to group social skills training', *Social Work With Groups*, 6, 3–4: 51–66.

Garvin, C.D. and Reed, B.G. (1983) 'Gender issues in social group work: an overview', *Social Work With Groups*, 6, 3–4: 5–18.

Garvin, C.D. and Reed, B.G. (1994) 'Small group theory and social work practice: promoting diversity and social justice', in Greene, R.R. (ed.) *Human Behaviour Theory: A Diversity Framework*, New York: Aldine de Gruyter.

Garvin, C.D. and Reed, B.G. (1995) 'Sources and visions for feminist group work: reflective processes, social justice, diversity, and connection', in Van Den Bergh, N. (ed.) *Feminist Practice in the 21st Century*, Washington, DC: NASW Press.

Gutiérrez, L. (1990) 'Working with women of color: an empowerment perspective', *Social Work*, 35, 2: 149–53.

Gutiérrez, L. and Lewis, E. (1999) *Empowering Women of Color*, New York: Columbia University Press.

Hanmer, J. and Statham, D. (1988) *Women and Social Work: Towards a Woman-Centred Practice*, Basingstoke: Macmillan, rev. edition 1998.

Healy, K. (2000) *Social Work Practices: Contemporary Perspectives on Change*, London: Sage.

Hirayama, J. and Hirayama, K. (1985) 'Empowerment through group participation: process and goal', in Parenes, M. (ed.) *Innovations in Social Group Work: Feedback from Practice to Theory*, Binghamton, NY: Haworth Press.

Holstein, B.B. and Laperdon-Addison, D. (1994) 'Groupwork for mental health providers utilising the enchanted self concept', *Groupwork*, 7, 2: 136–44.

Jones, M., Mordecai, M., Rutter, F. and Thomas, L. (1991) 'A Miskin model of groupwork with women offenders', *Groupwork*, 4, 3: 215–30.

Jordan, J.V., Kaplan, A.G., Miller, J.B., Stiver, I.P. and Surrey, J.L. (eds) (1991) *Women's Growth in Connection: Writings from the Stone Center*, New York: Guilford Press.

Kaufman, J. and Timmers, R.L. (1983) 'Searching for the hairy man', *Social Work With Groups*, 6, 3–4: 164–75.

Kent, R.L. and Moss, S.E. (1994) 'Effect of sex and gender on leadership: do traits matter?' *Academy of Management Executive*, 37: 1335–46.

Kolb, J.A. (1997) 'Are we still stereotyping leadership? A look at gender and other predictors of leader emergence', *Small Group Research*, 28, 3: 370–93.

Knight, C. (1990) 'Use of support groups with adult female survivors of child sexual abuse', *Social Work*, 35, 3: 202–6.

Krzowski, S. and Land, P. (eds) (1988) *In Our Experience: Workshops at the Women's Therapy Centre*, London: The Women's Press.

Leonard, P. (1997) *Postmodern Welfare: Reconstructing an Emancipatory Project*, London: Sage.

Lovell, M.L., Reid, K. and Richey, C.A. (1992) 'Social support training for abusive mothers', *Social Work With Groups*, 15, 2–3: 95–107.

Masson, H. and Erooga, M. (1990) 'The forgotten parent: groupwork with mothers of sexually abused children', *Groupwork*, 3, 2: 144–56.

Miller, S., Exner, T.M., Williams, S.P. and Ehrhardt, A.A. (2000) 'A gender specific intervention for at-risk women in the USA', *AIDS Care*, 12, 4: 603–13.

Mistry, T. (1989) 'Establishing a feminist model of groupwork in the probation service', *Groupwork*, 2, 2: 145–58.

Mistry, T. and Brown, A. (1991) 'Black/white co-working in groups', *Groupwork*, 4, 2: 101–18.

Mistry, T. and Brown, A. (eds) (1997) *Race and Groupwork*, London: Whiting & Birch.

Morson, T. and McInnis, R. (1983) 'Sexual identity issues in group work: gender, social sex role, and sexual orientation', *Social Work With Groups*, 6, 3–4: 67–77.

Muir, L. and Notta, H. (1993) 'An Asian mothers' group', *Groupwork*, 6, 2: 122–31.

Mullender, A. (1996) 'Groupwork with male "domestic" abusers', *Groupwork*, 9, 1: 27–47.

Mullender, A. and Ward, D. (1991) *Self-Directed Groupwork: Users Take Action for Empowerment*, London: Whiting & Birch.

Norman, C. (1994) 'Groupwork with young mothers', *Groupwork*, 7, 3: 223–35.

Otway, O. (1993) 'Art therapy: creative groupwork for women', *Groupwork*, 6, 3: 211–20.

Otway, O. and Peake, A. (1994) 'Using a facilitated self help group for women whose children have been sexually abused', *Groupwork*, 7, 2: 153–62.

Parton, N. and O'Byrne, P. (2000) *Constructive Social Work: Towards a New Practice*, Basingstoke: Macmillan.

Pease, B. and Fook, J. (eds) (1999) *Transforming Social Work Practice: Postmodern Critical Perspectives*, London: Routledge.

Pence, E. (1993) *Education Groups for Men Who Batter: The Duluth Model*, New York: Springer.

Raja, S. (1998) 'Culturally sensitive therapy for women of color', *Women and Therapy*, 21, 4: 67–84.

Reed, B.G. and Garvin, C. (eds) (1983) *Groupwork with Women/Groupwork with Men: An Overview of Gender Issues in Social Groupwork Practices*, Binghamton, New York: Haworth Press (published concurrently as *Social Work With Groups*, 6, 3–4).

Reid, K., Mathews, G. and Liss, P.S. (1995) 'My partner is hurting: group work with male partners of adult survivors of sexual abuse', *Social Work With Groups*, 18, 1: 81–7.

Rhode, D.L. (1989) *Justice and Gender: Sex Discrimination and the Law*, Cambridge, MA: Harvard University Press. (quoted in Figueira-McDonough *et al.* 1989).

Rhule, C. (1988) 'A group for white women with black children', *Groupwork*, 1, 1: 41–7.

Russell, M.N. (1995) *Confronting Abusive Beliefs: Group Treatment for Abusive Men*, Thousand Oaks, CA: Sage.

Saulnier, C.F. (2000) 'Incorporating feminist theory into social work practice: group work examples', *Social Work With Groups*, 23, 1: 5–29.

Schiller, L.Y. (1995) 'Stages of development in women's groups: a relational model', in Kurland, R. and Salmon, R. (eds) *Group Work Practice in a Troubled Society*, Binghamton, NY: Haworth Press.

Schiller. L.Y. (1997) 'Rethinking stages of development in women's groups', *Social Work With Groups*, 20, 3: 2–19.

Sharf, B.F. (1997) 'Communicating breast cancer on-line: support and empowerment on the internet', *Women and Health*, 26, 1: 65–84.

Shimanoff, S.B. and Jenkins, M.M. (1991) 'Leadership and gender: challenging assumptions and recognizing resources', in Cathcart, R.S. and Samovar, L.A. (eds) *Small Group Communication: A Reader*, Dubuque: William C. Brown.

Thompson, N. (1998) *Promoting Equality: Challenging Discrimination and Oppression in the Human Services*, Basingstoke: Macmillan.

Trevithick, P. (1995) '"Cycling over Everest": groupwork with depressed women', *Groupwork*, 8, 1: 5–33.

Tribe, R. and Shackman, J. (1989) 'A way forward: a group for refugee women', *Groupwork*, 2, 2: 159–66.

Van Nostrand, C.H. (1993) *Gender-Responsible Leadership: Detecting Bias, Implementing Interventions*, Newbury Park, CA: Sage.

Ward, D. (1998) 'Groupwork', in Adams, R., Dominelli, L. and Payne, M. (eds) *Social Work: Themes, Issues and Critical Debates*, Basingstoke: Macmillan.

White, M. (1988–89) 'The externalising of the problem and the reauthoring of lives and relationships', *Dulwich Centre Newsletter*, summer: 3–21. (Published in Adelaide, Australia.)

White, M. (1991) 'Deconstruction and therapy', *Dulwich Centre Newsletter*, 3: 21–40. (Published in Adelaide, Australia.)

White, V. (1995) 'Commonality and diversity in feminist social work', *British Journal of Social Work*, 25, 2: 143–56.

Williams, F. (1996) 'Postmodernism, feminism and the question of difference', in Parton, N. (ed.) *Social Theory, Social Change and Social Work*, London: Routledge.

Wintram, C. (ed.) (1994) 'Groupwork with women', special issue of *Groupwork*, 7, 2. (Whole issue)

Wintram, C., Chamberlain, K., Kuhn, M. and Smith, J. (1994) 'A time for women: an account of a group for women on an out of city housing development in Leicester', *Groupwork*, 7, 2: 125–35.

Women in MIND (1986) *Finding Our Own Solutions: Women's Experience of Mental Health Care*, London: MIND (National Association for Mental Health).

Chapter 2

Women's group development from a relational model and a new look at facilitator influence on group development

Linda Yael Schiller

Introduction

Group development is one of the most interesting aspects of working with groups of all types. There are a number of variables that influence stages of development in groups, including the presenting problem or group focus, the age, ethnicity, race, and gender of the members, environmental factors, and experience with groups – both of the members and of the facilitators. In addition, the facilitators' philosophy, stance or orientation to group work inevitably influences their choice of intervention and may also have an influence on how the group actually develops. Taking all these variables into account is important when planning and facilitating groups. This chapter focuses on the variable of gender, specifically of women's groups, but also beginning to explore related lessons for mixed groups and some men's groups.

The relational model of group development formulated by the author (Schiller 1995, 1997) examines how women's groups frequently seem to develop differently than the traditional models of group development would suggest. This relational model of group work is based on the work on women's psychological development arising out of the Stone Center for Research on Women at Wellesley College and at the Harvard Center for Gender Research at Harvard University. Miller (1976; see also Miller and Stiver 1991) and Gilligan (1982) examined the different developmental pathways that girls follow, the need for a differential understanding of the psychology of women and girls, and the subsequent changes practitioners need to make when working from this paradigm. This theoretical work provided a radical critique of male-dominated theoretical approaches to human development and suggested important implications for group development.

Having a coherent framework for group development is key for a group worker. Without a framework within which to understand expected and normative developments in the life of a group, workers would be at a loss to choose appropriate interventions that would both support where the members are at any given period of time and help the group to move forward to accomplish the goals and tasks of the members and of the group as a whole. If one recognizes the tasks and challenges at each group stage, and then assesses what is going on for the members at that given moment, the worker can choose a response that is timely. For example, if a group of women with a history of being abused is in the stage of establishing a relational base, the worker should probably not yet be encouraging the members to directly confront one another on issues or dilemmas. It is not yet the time to confront one another on how to handle other family members (e.g. "You should take him to court, what's the matter with you!"), because the members have not yet reached that stage of group development where they can safely do so without threatening the life of the group or the feelings of belonging and connectedness so crucial for healing. Rather, interventions should focus on establishing the felt sense of safety and furthering the bonds of support, connection, and affiliation so that members can later deal with the conflict in a safe and productive manner. If conflict does arise spontaneously, the worker certainly cannot simply ignore it, but will choose a different approach to it than in subsequent stages.

Understanding stages of group development is key for working with any population. To this end, reviewing some of the other prominent models of group development is useful, both because of their inherent value and because they can then serve as a basis of comparison with the relational model. What is interesting to observe across all of these other models, is that they assume conflict precedes intimacy, in contrast to what seems to happen in many women's groups where connection and affiliation through both similarities and differences not only precede overt expressions of conflict, but are necessary prerequisites for its productive resolution.

Review of other models of group development

One of the primary formulations in the field of social work in which the developmental course of groups has been charted has been the five stages of what has come to be known as the "Boston model." The work of Garland *et al.* (1965) became a standard format in which group development was described. The relational model of group work is based on a variation of this framework. Garland *et al.* (1965) outline five stages of development for groups:

1 pre-affiliation
2 power and control
3 intimacy
4 differentiation and
5 separation/termination.

Each stage has its own dynamic themes, its own inherent issues and struggles, and its own implications for facilitator interventions.

First, pre-affiliation is the time when members are trying to decide if this is really the group for them, with issues of trust and preliminary commitment at the foreground. Dynamic themes of approach/avoidance are common. The second stage, power and control, is described as a universal time of status jockeying for positions of power and for roles within the group structure. It is seen as a time when members challenge the authority of the group facilitator, a time of testing limits and boundaries, and a time of competition and challenge among members. Once having sufficiently resolved this normative crisis, members are free to move on to the third stage, intimacy, when mutuality and affiliation become the norm, when risk taking and self-disclosure are more evident and interpersonal connections deepen. In this model, the fourth stage, differentiation, is a time of greater self-expression and mutual support, of a higher degree of group cohesiveness, and a more reality-based recognition of the individuals comprising the group (including the facilitator). Finally, the fifth stage, separation, involves dealing with the impending loss of the group, a stage with some inherent anxiety, denial, recapitulation, review, evaluation, a time for letting go and separating.

Tuckman's work (1965) appears in the psychology literature. He also proposed a five-stage formulation of group development. Coining the stage names "forming," "storming," "norming," and "performing," (the term "adjourning," was added in 1977 by Tuckman and Jensen, to refer to the final ending or "mourning" stage). Tuckman (1965) described these stages as

1 testing and dependence
2 intragroup conflict
3 development of group cohesiveness and
4 functional role relatedness.

Tuckman (1965: 396) elaborates by explaining that, in the first stage, "groups initially concern themselves with orientation accomplished primarily through testing. Coincident with testing is the establishment of a dependent relationship on the leaders, other members, or preexisting standards." The second stage is characterized by conflict, resistance, and polarization around interpersonal issues. The third stage, group cohesiveness, develops when conflict and resistance are overcome and intimate personal feelings can be expressed. For Tuckman, the fourth stage, functional role relatedness, is seen as the time when "roles become flexible and functional," the group becomes a problem-solving entity, and solutions and insights emerge (1965: 396). Later on, in a review of the existing literature and research, Tuckman and Jensen (1977) added the fifth stage, termination.

Tuckman (1965: 396) also states that, although his suggested sequence can be seen across a variety of conditions of group life and composition, it "must be assumed that there is a finite range of conditions beyond which this sequence of development is altered," that, in other words, it may not be universal. This model, like that of Garland *et al.*, shares the orientation of conflict preceding cohesiveness and intimacy. (See also Bion 1961.)

Review of feminist theoretical underpinnings

A contrast to this literature is provided by the newer field of feminist theory and development, with its consequent impact on group work. The previously discussed formulations of group development were either constructed by men and/or based on the work and discussions of male theorists. It is important to review the history of recent feminist innovations in developmental theory to see their impact on group work.

Starting with Miller (1976), feminist theorists and practitioners began to explore the importance of relational development in framing a woman's sense of self in the world. Miller noted the centrality of connection and affiliation for women, in contrast to the traditional theories of psychological development which stressed increasing independence and autonomy as the necessary hallmarks of growth and adult mental health. Subsequent work by Gilligan (1982) continued to explore the centrality of attachment and connection for a woman's sense of self, and how this basic experience of connectedness in the world profoundly influences a woman's approach to conflict, disagreement and confrontation.

A collaboration by women at the Stone Center at Wellesley College during the 1970s developed a model of women's development called "self-in-relation" theory. Surrey (1991) has described the five main components of this model:

1   The deepening capacity for relationship and relational competence is a primary developmental goal. Other aspects of self, such as creativity, autonomy, and self assertion, emerge within the context of relationship, without needing to disconnect or sacrifice the relationship for self-development.
2   Empathy is a crucial feature. According to Surrey (1991) and Jordan (1991), there is a focus on mutuality and mutual empathy. Miller and Stiver (1991) describe mutuality in the therapeutic relationship as related to emotional authenticity. Empathic attunement includes balancing the affective and the cognitive components of a situation in order to accurately identify with another's feeling state.
3   The parent–child relationship is seen as the paradigm, or model, for other relationships. The strengths and weaknesses of this primary relationship often greatly influence the capacity or ability to engage in other relationships in life. Mutuality can occur as parent and child mirror each other and give to each other.
4   The basic developmental task is relationship-differentiation. Differentiation of self takes place *within*, not after, instead of, or outside of, the context of the relationship itself.
5   Relational authenticity is valued. It is defined as the challenge to feel emotionally real and connected in relationships. It includes risk, conflict, and expression of the full range of affects.

The language of the relational model is that of connection and disconnection. Everyone yearns for connection. Yet the paradox is that when a person has repeatedly met with disconnection in their past (e.g. withdrawal, abandonment, trauma, abuse, neglect, depression, hostility, loss, etc.), they may become so afraid of engaging that they develop techniques to stay out of connection. Shame frequently accompanies disconnection.

Issues of oppression and the use of an empowerment model of group practice are inextricably linked. The relational model of psychological development, and the adaptation of some of its principles for group work, have as their core premise the notion of righting the imbalances created by living in an oppressive culture. The relational concepts of mutuality, interpersonal empathy, and the sharing of power are antithetical to the perpetuation of oppression.

Shulman (1992: 35) describes the key concept of oppression psychology as "repeated exposure to oppression, subtle or direct, [which] may lead vulnerable members of an oppressed group to internalize the negative self images projected by the external oppressor." The combination of this internalized self-image and the repressed rage associated with the oppression (whether subtle or direct) may raise the threshold for vulnerable members to engage in destructive behaviors against themselves or others; thus participating in the oppression as auto-oppressors.

Many women describe a deep sense of shame in their lives that influences many of their actions and decisions. For example, one member of a women's writing group experienced a great deal of difficulty in writing an autobiographical piece that was to be presented at a public reading. She struggled with the idea that anything that she might have to say or, more specifically, anything that had happened to her in her life might have meaning or relevance to others. Margaret said, "I just can't bear the thought of others hearing me read about my own life. If this were a fictional piece, it wouldn't be such a problem. I really wish that others could relate to my experiences, but I'm sure that they can't. I'm afraid that they'll just think that it was stupid, or laugh at me."

If members of our groups have developed this sense of shame, it seems that they would need a great deal of safety before feeling free to venture outside of the small box they have enclosed themselves in for protection. Also striking in oppression psychology is the aspect of repressed rage. Externalizing this rage may lead to group behaviors of greater conflict early on, while internalizing the rage leads to the phenomenon of "niceness" we see in some women's groups, or in any group where the facilitator is not able to work through their own personal relationship with conflict and utilize their group work skills to facilitate a safe and productive outlet for the anger.

Providing an antidote to feelings of shame, loss of voice, and negative self-images is what an empowerment perspective attempts to accomplish. According to Gutiérrez (1990: 149), empowerment is "a process of increasing personal, interpersonal, or political power so the individuals can take action to improve their life circumstances." Rappaport, as quoted in Gutiérrez (1990), describes empowerment as indicating a sense of control over one's own life. The process of empowerment occurs when the person is able to develop a sense of personal power, an ability to affect others, and an ability to work with others to effect change.

The empowerment literature describes group work as the ideal modality for empowering practice (Gutiérrez 1990; Mullender and Ward 1991). Gutiérrez describes an empowering practice as a helping relationship based on collaboration, trust, and the sharing of power. These are also the cornerstones of group work based on the relational model of group development. This model moves from its earliest pre-affiliation stage directly into relationship building and establishing a sense of trust and safety (rather than addressing issues of conflict first, as is the norm of most other models). Only then does this paradigm encourage venturing on to the challenge of re-learning how to maintain relationships in the face of both difference and conflict. Many women lose a sense of personal power in the face of oppressive and patriarchal cultural norms, as well as in the specifics of neglect, abuse, loss, or shaming in their own lives. To help them to become re-empowered, it makes sense to work with women in groups in a way that starts with what they already do well, and then move on to encourage growth by staying connected through differences and through overt conflict.

The place of conflict in the relational model of group development

The relational model (Schiller 1995) suggests a paradigm for stages of development in women's groups that incorporates the growing body of recent feminist scholarship on women's growth and development and takes into account the forces of oppression and silencing in women's lives. Attending to the centrality of connection and affiliation, women's need for a felt sense of safety in a group, and their different relationships with power and conflict, my proposed sequence of normative development for women's groups looks as follows:

1 pre-affiliation
2 establishing a relational base
3 mutuality and interpersonal empathy
4 challenge and change
5 separation and termination.

One of the contrasts with more traditional models is that conflict occurs much later in women's groups, not immediately following pre-affiliation as power and control or "storming." Affiliative strivings come sooner and safe connections are necessary prerequisites for the later emergence of productive conflict. It would seem that the ability to comfortably hold power and to engage in conflict are the cutting edges of growth for many women, while engaging in deep empathic connection is the growth edge for many men.

Stage two of the relational model, establishing a relational base, is a time when women come together to form bonds of affiliation and connection and establish the felt sense of safety in the group that will enable them to later move into the more challenging activities of dealing with conflict. This is in contrast to Garland *et al.* (1965), who view the second stage as a time when conflict is high and which involves status and power jockeying, tests of limits and boundaries, challenge to authority, and interpersonal challenges and competition.

An example of establishing a relational base occurred in a group for abused women who had left their partners. During their second and third meetings they spent a great deal of time comparing notes on what had allowed them to make the decision to leave, and what they were doing to try to enhance their safety now. Many of them discovered that perceiving a growing threat to their children was a common theme that helped them take the risk to leave.

The third stage of mutuality incorporates elements both of intimacy and of differentiation, moving beyond simple connection and recognition of sameness to a stage of mutuality that allows for both empathic connection and for difference. While not yet engaged in overt conflict or challenges at this stage, members are able to allow and appreciate each other's differences within the framework of their affiliation and connection. This again is in contrast to Garland *et al.* (1965), who separate the stages of intimacy and differentiation. If the members have successfully negotiated the first two stages, they can now hold on to their differences without worrying about losing the authenticity or genuineness of the relationships in the process.

An example of this stage was provided by an infertility group. All of the women joining the group had been trying to get pregnant for at least a year. Initially, their relief at being "in the same boat" (Shulman 1992: 276) was high, and members spent time comparing their common struggles and giving each other support. As time went on and the group moved into the third stage, mutuality, some of the women in the group began to get pregnant, while others did not. Now difference in circumstance became quite highlighted, yet the women were able to continue the connections they had forged in the face of these differences.

The fourth stage is that of challenge and change. The challenge in this stage is often at the heart of growth for women: how to engage in and negotiate conflict without sacrificing the bonds of connection and empathy in doing so. It is here that members can confront themselves, the facilitators, other members. Fedele (1994: 7) describes a relational approach to managing conflict in a group as one in which "a context of safety and empathy has been created . . . that can contain divergent realities even when they conflict . . . and that keeps the experience of anger within the connection." Fedele's formulation regarding managing conflict nicely summarizes the ideal outcome of work done in stages two and three, during which the tools are built that can then be used to negotiate this fourth stage.

An example of this stage occurred in a group for mothers of children who had been sexually abused. The norm which had emerged in the group was that of expressing only anger or outrage at the offenders, whether or not the members had a relationship with them prior to the disclosure of the abuse. After the group had been meeting for nine months, Jody revealed that she had visited her husband in prison; an announcement that she was fairly certain would not be received favorably by the rest of the group. As she had predicted, the rest of the members initially pounced on her. Jody spoke of her ambivalence about completely letting go of what had been a positive relationship prior to the disclosure of abuse. Eventually, other members in the group were able to redirect the anger they initially focused on Jody to its more appropriate repository, the perpetrators.

The role of the facilitator in group development

The literature of group work has long approached the concept of group development by describing what is happening in the phases of groups, formulating theories to explain these stages, and then applying knowledge of this theory to actual interventions in groups. When working with a coherent theory base that describes the actual behavior of groups, it all fits rather nicely. The key is, did work get done? If so, then the group is working appropriately for its multivariable components.

When, on the other hand, the theory doesn't seem to fit what is actually happening in our groups, there are several choices. One is to see whether, for reasons of group composition, environmental factors, facilitator experience, or other factors, the group may have gotten stuck at a particular point. It may then need some intervention to get it moving along.

A second choice is to decide that what we are seeing is not just an anomaly; that our group seems to be working in a manner that suits its members even though it doesn't mesh with theory as we know it. We can formulate a different theoretical base. The relational model of group development arose from the author's experience in the field, supported by other practitioners of women's groups that also failed to follow the existing paradigm yet seemed to be functioning well and getting work done within an alternative framework.

A third option is to examine what the facilitator is bringing to the group in the form of style, orientation, philosophy, and theoretical base, and to see if that itself may be influencing what is happening in the group. We are used to looking at stages of group development from a descriptive basis; it may be that we can look at them from a proactive basis as well. We need to remember that, as Kelly and Berman-Rossi (2000) state, group development models describe what might happen, not what should happen. To do this opens up theoretical and ethical questions. What is the influence of the facilitator on how the group moves along, how it works, how it resolves its dilemmas, and how it deals with the omnipresent themes of intimacy and authority described by Shulman (1992) and others? If we approach our group from a particular stance, what will that do to the actual evolution of the life-cycle of the group? For example, if we come from a relational stance that emphasizes the centrality and importance of connection, continuity and mutuality in relationships, and the need for a strong relational holding space before delving deeply into conflict, what will that do to the evolving culture and development of the group? The shift in this line of thinking when examining the relational model of group development moves from how the group organically develops to an examination of how the worker may actually influence this process by his/her own presence and style.

One example of the possible influence of worker stance in promoting a relational model of group development can be seen in a classroom seminar on sexual minorities described by DeLois and Cohen (2000). This classroom group was composed of both men and women, although women were the clear majority (fourteen to one). The worker/professor facilitated a very rapid development of a relational model in several ways:

- She made clear her own predisposition to the relational model of group work from the outset.
- She made personal self-disclosures relevant to the purpose of the group early on, thus modeling the stages both of establishing a relational base and of mutuality and interpersonal empathy (connections through similarities and establishing a safe space, and a non-hierarchical facilitative style).
- She used the development of the group contract to enhance a group culture that evolved along the lines of the relational model by stressing early connections, followed by a stress on mutuality through differences, and then rules on safety, tolerance, respect and empathy.

While many of these are part of standard group contracting, they also set a tone early on for the examination of conflict within a framework of connection, foreshadowing the fourth stage, challenge and change.

In an even more overtly prescriptive fashion, Sternbach (2001) describes using the group work model of relational theory to facilitate his men's groups. Here, all the members as well as the facilitators are men, yet Sternbach is in favor of workers utilizing the relational model to help men to heal in the arenas in which they have typically had more difficulty than women, those of forming and maintaining close intimate connections that can contain personal self-disclosure and risk taking. He describes his groups as developing along the lines of the stages of development of the relational model, which may seem contrary to expectation for men's groups. The clear differentiating factor was the worker's orientation and encouragement.

We then return to the social work paradigm of group work with its quandary for the facilitator between "following " and "leading" in our groups. Clearly there are times when we do both, and when it may be ethical and professional group work practice to do one or the other. However, given the state of our knowledge, and the inherent power resting in us as practitioners, it is imperative that we examine and are cognizant of our values and predispositions as group workers, for they will affect our groups. We thus need to be aware of our own orientations in order to practice ethically and without hidden agendas. We constantly monitor ourselves and make judgement calls as to when to go with the flow of an organically evolving group culture or direction of the moment, and when to lend a vision, as Schwartz (1961) encouraged us to do, in moving the group towards another way of working together – as indicated to us by our experience of group work, of that particular group's needs given its context and population, and by our own philosophical bent.

We need to attend not only to what we are looking for but also to what we are ignoring; not only to what we are encouraging, but to what we are discouraging; not only to what we are stating overtly, but also to what we are implying covertly. For example, a flier publicised a workshop on group work entitled "The nice group and group leaders' avoidance of conflict and the need for approval." Clearly this speaker experienced herself and other female group facilitators as having both the same affiliative needs as the members and the same desire to "make nice" and avoid conflict. Her premise was that the group facilitator colludes in maintaining a friendly atmosphere at the cost of ignoring the group's needs to begin the process of challenge and change. We need to examine and be conscious of our theoretical base as well as pay attention to any feelings that arise in the context of doing the work. As women facilitating groups, in addition to resonating with universal feelings of loss that come up irrespective of the manifest content and purpose of the group we need to be particularly aware of our own relationship with conflict and anger, and of any strategies we ourselves have developed to avoid it. Mark Twain is reported to have said that, when the only tool you have is a hammer, the whole world looks like a nail. We need to make sure that we have as many tools of our trade as possible in our repertoire, and that we use them with care and a differential approach.

Implications for practice

Using examples from the world of practice, this section further explores the middle three stages that differentiate this model from others. Implicit in working with a phased model of group development is that, not only are facilitators looking for different group behaviors at different stages of development, but also that we have a role in eliciting them. We make choices about interventions throughout the life of the group. We must bring to our groups a well-grounded knowledge base of group work principles, some specific experience or at least substantial research about the specifics of our population, context and presenting concerns, and an awareness of our own process, our biases and beliefs, and our responses. Being informed and cognizant of our practice base will guide us in deciding how and when to intervene, when to remain silent, when and how to encourage the members to delve into the appropriate layer of work, and when to redirect or suggest an alternative option. Having supervision or consultation is critical for both new and seasoned workers.

It is important to remember that stages of group development are not universally linear. Particularly in open-ended groups, where the norm is the coming and going of members, an individual member may be at a different stage of her group process than is the group as a whole, depending on her length of time in the group. The group as a whole may also experience ebbs and flows in its process of working, as it deals with the addition or loss of one of its members or if a particularly thorny issue prompts a return to use of strategies for disconnection rather than of empathic resonance or attunement. A caveat to facilitator intervention at different group stages is to also take into account these vicissitudes in individual members and their abilities to form connection, to tolerate differences, and to deal with conflict productively. Berman-Rossi (1993) reminds us to individualize our work for each group, using a multivariable consciousness of such factors as the race, gender, ethnicity, age, class, and focus of the group. That said, there are still worker orientations and intervention choices at each stage of development that can optimally promote movement and growth.

Notably, in the second stage of establishing a relational base, the worker can help to promote connection and the beginnings of empathic attunement by encouraging members to find their points of connection and actively helping members to establish a safe space. Rather than being on the lookout for issues of status, jockeying for position, or shifting power dynamics associated with the power and control stage, workers can tune in to themes of affiliation, similarity, and safety. Articulating the process as members find commonalities, and making explicit that this is a healthy and valued process, are two key facilitator roles. Certainly, if some kind of conflict should arise at this stage it needs to be addressed, but encouraging engagement in conflict, disagreement, or expression of anger is not a facilitator role at this stage.

An example from a group at a women's residential substance abuse center is described by Bertolotti (2000). We can see in this example that the two facilitators did not share a similar orientation, and that their interventions to the same stimulus were quite different, evoking different responses from the group. During the group check-in, Judy said that there wasn't much going on and she didn't have much to share. It was clear to the facilitators, however, that something was bothering her. One facilitator confronted her, saying that she thought there was something going on, and Judy began to cry, saying she felt too ashamed to talk to the group. The other facilitator looked around at the group and said that everyone was here to support her, and that everyone was struggling with similar issues in their lives and their sobriety. The members added their support, and said that they were there for her, not to judge her. Judy then admitted that while she was out on an overnight pass she became very drunk and passed out on the bathroom floor, where her son found her. The other members responded empathically, hugged her and cried with her, and shared their own struggles with urges to drink or use drugs.

In this example we can see that the premature confrontation or challenge by one facilitator backfired, while, by attending to the need for safety, support, and similarity of circumstance and struggle, the other facilitator allowed the member to feel safe enough in her vulnerability to make an important self-disclosure.

Time is needed to develop a sense of safety in this stage. Because of a history of general disempowerment (Miller 1976), as well as specific histories of violence or threat, workers must never take for granted that the women in a group feel safe. Developing a contract together with the group that highlights these issues is one strategy to enhance safety. For example, in a group of adult survivors of sexual abuse, the contract was developed together with the members and recorded on a chart which was hung on the wall each week thereafter. Elements discussed in detail and recorded included issues around no touching without explicit permission, no sexual contact ever between members or facilitators, what safety talismans could be brought to group, and the whole issue of confidentiality. The traditional injunction, "what is said in group stays in group," was explored, as also were the difference between confidentiality and secrets, the issues of trust and the relational rupture of that trust as a result of the abuse, and what to do if they ran into each other outside of group. Near the end of the group, when a member wanted a commemorative photograph taken, the contract around confidentiality was revisited as members discussed the pros and cons of this and what guidelines would ensure this felt safe. They ultimately decided that it would be OK to take the picture, a decision they were able to come to because of the high attention to safety established as a basic group guideline (see Schiller and Zimmer 1994).

The third stage of this model is marked by the emergence of mutuality and interpersonal empathy, both among and between the members, and between the facilitator and the members. Workers can make conscious choices to promote an empowering "power with" rather than an oppressive "power over" atmosphere (Miller 1976). There are several ways in which a facilitator may do this. One is to engage in a non-hierarchical style of facilitation, in which making brilliant interpretations is abandoned in favor of the member-as-expert stance. While the worker can certainly add her insights or opinions, it is not assumed by either the worker or the members that the worker has the final word.

An interesting example of this process is from a dream circle group meeting. Here members come together with a facilitator for the purpose of working on understanding their dreams and learning to use their dream insights for their personal and/or professional lives. The whole premise of the group's experience of working together on an individual's dream is that the only one who has the final say on an interpretation or insight is the dreamer. Only when the dreamer has the "Aha!" feeling is it a fit. Working with dreams is, by definition, an intimate experience, and this stage of empathic connection combined with respect for differences is often swiftly reached. In one member's dream, there was a tree that contained a great deal of interest and energy for her. Opinions offered by the facilitator and the members ranged from the tree being a symbol of growth, to the dreamer needing to change direction in life ("barking up the wrong tree"), to a spiritual connection as the tree was rooted in the earth and also reaching up to the heavens, to a connection with the member's childhood when she had frequently retreated to sit with a book in a tall tree in her yard. There was no differentiation made between the "rightness" of one meaning over another, or between those offered by members or by the facilitator. The final answer lay with the member whose dream it was.

A related issue is the importance of the worker letting the group know when he or she has been emotionally moved by the group. So many people have experienced relationship disconnections where they were unable to reach the other person or they did not know if they were having any effect on the lives of others. Therefore, feedback that honors and acknowledges the member's ability to connect and have an impact is crucial. Relational authenticity and presence by the worker help to create a relational context for empowerment of the members and a greater willingness to risk sharing from a deeper self. Authenticity in responding to member impact can be a factor in helping the group to move. It can also model the ability to simultaneously hold power and authority and to relate and react from a place of empathic attunement, a combination that many women may not have experienced in their lives outside of group.

Co-facilitation presents an opportunity for workers to model the collaboration and cooperation within the authority and power for group members, thus providing an *in vivo* experience for group members to see the two facilitators work with both their similarities and their differences in style, orientation, temperament, and affect (Leveillee 2000). When two facilitators can respect each other's differences and still share the power inherent in their role, there can be a profound effect on the members' own abilities to do so.

Finally, the stage of challenge and change may provide members and workers alike with the opportunity to find their own voice and to stay connected in spite not only of differences but of outright expressions of disagreement, anger, and conflict. The progression then becomes the ability to stay connected through similarities, through differences, and through conflict. When a group of professional women were asked to identify associations with the word "conflict," those that emerged were: "avoid it," "bad," "scarey," "make nice," "hostility," "opportunity," "stomach ache," "anxiety," "fear." Only one word in the list, "opportunity," suggested anything positive. So it is imperative that facilitators examine their own associations and reactions to the work needing to be done at this stage so that they don't unwittingly let their personal responses impede the group. The challenge for facilitators is to not only allow, but even to use and, at times, encourage the rough-edged energy of conflict, anger, and disagreement without attempting to smooth it out or "make nice" too quickly. If the group has successfully negotiated the earlier stages of connecting and of respecting and holding difference within connection, they are now ready and able to hold connection within conflict as well. The facilitator will help the group to integrate the aggression and to use the energy for assertion, growth, and change. Conflict needs to be reframed as containing the potential for growth.

This fourth stage may also be a time when workers need to step up their active interventions in the group for a time, rather than become less active, as in previous models of group work. Garland *et al.* (1965), Tuckman (1965), and others, see this fourth stage as a time when the group has resolved most of its issues about working together, so that the worker role is more observational and less interventive. It may be that, in women's groups, with the more direct attention to conflict emerging now, the worker needs to play a more prominent role as the members begin to grapple directly with the very areas that are the most difficult. Members may need additional support in dealing directly with content and also in reflecting on their process and way of working together at this time. Directly clarifying that this work on conflict, anger, and confrontational skills is a key part of their personal and collective growth process can help remove some of the fears and anxieties that are bound to be present when taking risks. Assuring members that the worker's job at this juncture is to help them stay connected and not lose their relationships as they do this work can be very comforting, and it can reinforce that this is a safe place to try out new behaviors. This role of the worker may be key in allowing some groups to engage fully in this stage of development.

In one class on group work, which was run with attention to internal group process as well as to content, a member challenged both the professor/facilitator and his fellow classmates. The composition of the class was 80 per cent women, so this male member was in a minority in terms of gender, but also in terms of race, as he was of Hispanic background and the majority of the others were Caucasian. The class dynamics had developed along the lines of the relational model, due in part to composition and in part to facilitator orientation to that model. In the tenth session of a thirteen-week semester, Jorge challenged the class for not paying enough attention to racial issues and differences. He claimed that the previous discussions on that issue were too short and superficial, and that he was feeling short-changed as a result. The rest of the class initially sat in silence after his statements, although they were usually a lively group that didn't hesitate to participate without needing to be invited to do so. The facilitator thanked Jorge for raising his concern, and invited others to participate in a discussion by saying, "Let's take some time to respond to Jorge. It's clearly an important issue for us all, and it's fine to have a range of feelings and opinions about it." After this blatant invitation to respond, and to disagree if desired, the class members engaged in a lively discussion, including asking Jorge why he had waited before bringing this up, and others saying that they would often hold back from offering opinions because they were afraid to offend him or the other minority members in the class out of their own ignorance. We can see from this example that the facilitator did take a more active role in helping the members to engage in conflict, and that she not only implicitly reinforced this as a safe place in which to do so, but was inclusive of herself, using "us" rather than "you" in her wording.

Conclusion

Working from a relational model of group development gives group workers an opportunity to match their facilitation style with the developmental needs of their groups. The primacy of connection and affiliation for women and the emergence of productive conflict later on in the life of the group are key components of this model. This discussion has highlighted the importance of using differential worker interventions at the different stages in the life of the group. Overt attention to the creation of a safe holding space and of mutuality that includes the worker, and the potential need for more active guidance by the worker when the group is ready to deal directly with conflict, have been emphasized as roles for the facilitator using this model. This framework grew out of experience with and observations of women's groups, though it may also be applicable to other groups, particularly those with vulnerable populations as their members. The discussion has also examined the potential influence the worker herself has on how the group develops, and the need both for cognizance of this dynamic and for authenticity about our own orientations as we approach our groups. We can be aware of the descriptive and the prescriptive potential of the stages of group development. The relational model can offer a powerful antidote to the forces of shame, oppression, and silencing that many women experience, and help members to regain their true voice.

References

Berman-Rossi, T. (1993) "The tasks and skills of the social worker across stages of group development," *Social Work With Groups*, 16, 1–2: 69–81.

Bertolotti, D. (2000) "Group process: connection as a healing force for women substance abusers," unpublished MSW paper.

DeLois, K. and Cohen, M.B. (2000) "A queer idea: using group work principles to strengthen learning in a sexual minorities seminar," *Social Work With Groups*, 23, 3: 53–67.

Fedele, N. (1994) *Relationships in Groups: Connection, Resonance, and Paradox*, Working Paper No. 69, Wellesley, MA: Stone Center for Research on Women, Wellesley College.

Garland, J., Jones, H., and Kolodny, R. (1965) "A model for stages of development in social work groups," in Bernstein, S. (ed.) *Exploration in Group Work: Essays in Theory and Practice*, Boston, MA: Boston University School of Social Work.

Gilligan, C. (1982) *In a Different Voice*, Cambridge, MA: Harvard University Press.

Gutiérrez, L. (1990) "Working with women of color: An empowerment perspective," *Social Work*, 35, 2: 149–153.

Jordan, J. (1991) "Empathy and self boundaries", in Jordan, J., Kaplan, A., Miller, J.B., Stiver, I. and Surrey, J. (eds) *Women's Growth and Connection*, New York, Guilford Press.

—— (1997) "A relational perspective for understanding women's development," in Jordan, J. (ed.) *Women's Growth in Diversity*, New York: Guilford Press.

Jordan, J., Kaplan, A., Miller, J.B., Stiver, I., and Surrey, J. (eds) (1991) *Women's Growth in Connection: Writings from the Stone Center*, New York: Guilford Press.

Kelly, T. and Berman-Rossi, T. (2000) "Advancing stages of group development theory: the case of institutionalized older persons," *Social Work With Groups*, 22, 2–3: 119–38.

Leveillee, C. (2000) "Differential group work: oppression, women, and domestic violence," unpublished MSW paper.

Miller, J.B. (1976) *Toward a New Psychology of Women*, Boston, MA: Beacon Press.

Miller, J.B. and Stiver, I. (1991) *A Relational Reframing of Therapy*, Working Paper No. 52, Wellesley, MA: Stone Center for Research on Women, Wellesley College.

Mullender, A. and Ward, D. (1991) *Self-Directed Groupwork: Users Take Action for Empowerment*, London: Whiting & Birch.

Schiller, L.Y. (1995) "Stages of development in women's groups: a relational model," in Kurland, R. and Salmon, R. (eds) *Group Work Practice in a Troubled Society*, New York: Haworth Press.

—— (1997) "Rethinking stages of development in women's groups: implications for practice," *Social Work With Groups*, 20, 3: 3–19.

Schiller, L.Y. and Zimmer, B. (1994) "Sharing the secrets: the power of women's groups for sexual abuse survivors," in Gitterman, A. and Shulman, L. (eds) *Mutual Aid Groups, Vulnerable Populations, and the Life Cycle*, New York: Columbia University Press.

Schwartz, W. (1961) "The social worker as change agent," in *The Social Welfare Forum*, New York: Columbia University Press.

Shulman, L. (1992) *The Skills of Helping Individuals, Families, and Groups*, Itasca, IL: Peacock Publishers.

Sternbach, J. (2001) "Men connecting and changing: stages of relational growth in men's groups," *Social Work With Groups*, 23, 4: 59–69.

Surrey, J. (1991) "The self in relation: a theory of women's development," in Jordan, J.,

Kaplan, A., Miller, J.B., Stiver, I. and Surrey, J. (eds) *Women's Growth in Connection: Writings from the Stone Center*, New York: Guilford Press.

Tuckman, B. (1965) "Developmental sequence in small groups," *Psychological Bulletin*, 63, 6: 384–99.

Tuckman, B. and Jensen, M.A. (1977) "Stages of small group development revisited," in *Group and Organizational Studies*, 2, 1: 419–17.

Chapter 3

Women in groups: the history of feminist empowerment

Marcia B. Cohen

Women and groups

Collectivity, as an integral part of feminist ideology (Bricker-Jenkins *et al.* 1991; Butler and Wintram 1991; Jordan *et al.* 1991), has led to a long-standing emphasis on opportunities for women to explore issues together in single-sex groups. Socialized as highly relational beings (Jordan *et al.* 1991), women have been seen as likely to prefer group contexts over potentially isolating individual interactions, at least for many endeavors and, though it would now be regarded as essentialist and as dichotomizing men and women, this has been regarded in practice as a difference between most women and most men. Chapter 5 of this volume, by Bob Pease, does seem to concur that men do not find it easy in groups to share things about themselves or their gender roles, although it also reveals that some men want to make the effort and that some such groups can succeed. Feminist women, on the other hand, have long recognized and articulated the need to progress from focusing on individual issues to address broader group concerns (Bricker-Jenkins *et al.* 1991; Saulnier 2000), and there have been extended and extensive efforts to make this happen (Butler and Wintram 1991).

Consciousness-raising in groups

This shift from the personal to the political was given voice in the widespread development and growth of consciousness-raising groups in the 1960s, when the second wave of feminism generated a strong international women's movement. Consciousness-raising groups emerged spontaneously and informally, providing a supportive medium within which women could express their pain and frustration, and their experiences of oppression in patriarchal marriages, families, communities, and societies. Consciousness-raising groups tended to be leaderless, eschewing the more hierarchical and formal structures of traditional male-oriented organizations in favor of a more egalitarian structure (Freeman 1970).

In the language of group work, these indigenous groups initially functioned as support and mutual-aid groups, addressing the personal and interpersonal concerns of women. The mutual-aid networks that developed were critically important for many women. The groups evolved, and, over time, turned to examine the larger patriarchal social structure, signifying the groups' increasing awareness of the interconnections between the personal and the political. As women began to confront the societal forces responsible for their oppression, consciousness-raising groups increasingly took on the functions of social action groups. Support and action groups spanning both of these purposes began to be developed by professionals in social agency settings – for example, domestic violence agencies, community drop-in centres, and programs for single mothers. Feminist social action groups represent an outgrowth from the early women's movement groups, in that they encompass personal, interpersonal, and political dimensions (Cohen and Mullender 1999).

Feminist social action groups

Feminist social action groups have been described as having roots in the activist social goals groups that emerged in the 1960s (Papell and Rothman 1966). The social goals model was refined and developed to incorporate feminist and empowerment practice theory and to emphasize the importance of member control, an anti-oppressive stance and a social change focus (Mullender and Ward 1991; Cohen 1994; Lee 1994; Breton 1995). It has also encompassed diversity (Gutiérrez and Lewis 1999). The role of feminist social action group workers included facilitating opportunities for the empowerment of group members, assisting them with the process of determining social action goals and strategies, aiding in the implementation of social action, and specifically challenging internal and external forms of oppression, particularly gender oppression.

Feminist social action group work was exemplified by the self-directed group work model developed by Mullender and Ward (1991). As detailed by the authors, self-directed group work targeted external goals identified by group members through a process which involved them in focusing, in turn, on *what* were the major problems in their lives, *why* these existed, and *how* to tackle them. Central to this approach were six practice principles:

- emphasizing the avoidance of labels;
- honouring the rights of group members;
- basing intervention on a power analysis;
- assisting people to attain collective power through coming together in groups;
- opposing oppression through practice; and
- group workers facilitating rather than leading.

These practice principles were drawn from a value base emanating out of socialist feminist ideology and a commitment to activism (among other influences), resting on a presupposed social structural analysis of the issues facing women and other oppressed groups. Systemic inequalities based on gender, race, ethnicity, class, sexual orientation, age, and ability were understood as being inherently disempowering to all but the most privileged groups in society, and hence supportive of an oppressive status quo (Mullender and Ward 1991).

Feminist social action groups did not have therapeutic purposes. Indeed, such groups sought to challenge the negative labeling of service users as a result of interventions that inappropriately intervened at the individual level. Nevertheless, while feminist social action groups were focused primarily on structural analysis and external change, positive personal and interpersonal changes could and did occur as a consequence of participation (Cohen and Mullender 1999). This integration of personal and interpersonal gains with broader social change goals was highly consistent with feminist ideology (Bricker-Jenkins *et al.* 1991; Butler and Wintram 1991; Gutiérrez and Lewis 1999; Saulnier 2000). While the facilitator of the self-directed group was, by definition, not directive, she was active in providing the necessary resources and skills to help the group define its goals and move from more personal concerns to political examination and social action. This non-hierarchical model of group facilitation fitted well with feminism and its emphasis on egalitarianism and empowerment (Saulnier 2000).

Oppression as a locus for practice

Feminist social action group work practice in that era recognized the inter-connectedness of many forms of oppression. Gender oppression was seen as being inextricably tied to other forms of marginalization and discrimination: notably classism, racism, heterosexism, ageism and ableism. The dominant population was regarded as maintaining its power by oppressing other groups. Historically, at least in the West, this took the form of upper-middle and upper-class Caucasian, Anglo-Saxon, able, heterosexual males wielding power at the expense of working-class and poor people, people of color, lesbian, gay, bisexual and transgendered people, disabled people and women.

Oppressed and marginalized people were seen as able to combat the power of the status quo only if they worked together with others who were similarly oppressed. Their power came from their ability to recognize their common objectives and act in alliance. They could draw strength from group membership, from the personal knowledge that they were not alone, the interpersonal experience of support and mutual aid with others in the same boat, and the solidarity and political power that derived from collective action.

By 1991, Bricker-Jenkins was suggesting that feminist practitioners not only accepted diversity but actively sought to incorporate an awareness of diversity into their work. Similarly, in her discussion of empowering practice with women of color, Gutiérrez stated that "small group work is . . . the ideal modality for empowering interventions" (Gutiérrez 1991: 205). Within the social action and self-directed group work traditions, it was quite consistent with the worker's role to promote group discussion of the parallel and interconnected impact of various forms of oppression in disempowering the many in order to sustain the power of the few. The liberating process of group members systematically examining what were the major problems in their lives, why these exist, and how to tackle them – central to self-directed groupwork (Mullender and Ward 1991) – could be particularly useful in generating in group members an understanding of the interconnectedness of the "isms" and developing strategies to combat them: personally, interpersonally, and through social action and change.

By 1999, Gutiérrez and Lewis were overwhelmingly emphasizing the importance of identifying, acknowledging, and validating diversity within the context of a single social grouping, so as to explore in an empowerment group context the interconnected impact of the "isms" (sexism, racism, classism, heterosexism, ageism and ableism). They emphasize the importance, too, of the professional group facilitator actively working to reduce power discrepancies between themselves and group members as an aspect of locating "bottom–up" power.

Now, as a result of postmodernism, it has become difficult to talk about "top–down" oppression or the search for universal justice, or about women as a homogeneous group or one that is dichotomized from men. Let us glance back over feminist social action practice to see what we might risk losing as a result of these theoretical advances, and what might be worth retaining within a more sophisticated analysis of gender, power and social change.

Practice examples

An abused women's group

A group for women in abusive relationships, held some years ago in a domestic violence agency in the US, illustrates a number of the strengths of feminist social action group work that encouraged group members to look to *themselves* for an understanding of their problems. All members of the group had been in oppressive, violent relationships, tacitly supported by the larger society which the group worker saw as privileging men over women. The group was unusual in the degree of its diversity, with members ranging from affluent to very poor, and including Caucasian, African-American, and Latina women; at the time, all identified as heterosexual.

As different as these women were, their commonalities drew them together. As group members examined the ways in which their husbands and boyfriends had controlled, demeaned, and disempowered them, they saw their own experiences reflected in each other's lives and began to see each other and themselves in terms of their strengths. The mutuality and connection in this group were powerful, and enabled them to analyse their individual and shared oppression in order to better understand and combat it.

Although the members of this group tended to emphasize their similarities – exclaiming, for example, "Our stories are so much alike, we must all be married to the same man!" – the facilitator encouraged them also to acknowledge and appreciate their differences. The following interchange between five group members demonstrates the interconnectedness between diversity, oppression, and role of empowerment and collective action:

Virginia (a Caucasian mother of two sons, not employed outside the home, whose husband was a bank vice-president): I don't know what to do! My husband changed all the bank accounts to just his name. He closed the safe deposit box, I have no money at all. He is using money to control me, to get me to do his bidding. Today I could not even buy groceries.

Lori (an African-American mother of three, on public assistance, whose boyfriend works sporadically): Honey, join the club! I could write the book about not having money for food. But you can't let him control you. You are used to having nice things, living in a nice house, driving a fancy car. But those are shackles, girl. Your dignity is more important than having nice furniture and cars and things. If you can find ways to manage without his money, then he can't control you so much.

Virginia: So, can you tell me how? How do I manage without his money? I don't know how to do it, I don't even know where to start!

Diane (an African-American woman, employed as a domestic, who had recently left her husband): First of all, if you leave him you can sue him for child support for your two kids. He is loaded, so you will do OK. In the meantime you can get public assistance, job training, food stamps. Today you should go to the food pantry at that church on Western Boulevard. They're only open on Mondays and Wednesdays, so make sure you get there this afternoon. That will tide you over until you get your benefits. The social worker here at the Women's Centre can help you apply.

Virginia: Wow! You know so much. Thanks. This is very new and scarey for me. I'm not even sure I am ready to leave Richard. I know I sound like a whiny, poor little rich white girl, but, I have always just taken care of the boys, kept the house up, and entertained Richard's clients. I have no job experience or skills. I have lived a sheltered life, now I am paying for it.

Denise (a single white woman college student, with an abusive boyfriend): I bet you have learned more from raising children and keeping house than you realize. (*Turning to the other three women*) Do you see the two of us as spoiled whiny white women?

Adela (a middle-aged, working-class Puerto Rican woman, living with an abusive husband): I don't see anyone here as whiny. A punch in the stomach hurts real bad whatever colour you are.

Lori: Adela is right. Sure you are white, Virginia, plus you are very rich. But what good has that done you? It is your husband who has the money, and he uses it to keep you down. I may be black and poor, and that makes my life harder than yours in many ways, but in some ways I have more freedom than you. I have always been poor and always had to take care of myself. I guess I have learned how to do it pretty well. I may get hit, but at least I can fight back in some ways, subtle like . . .

Following that interchange, the facilitator asked if any of the others felt they could fight back and, if so, how. This led to a broader discussion of the ways in which women, poor people, and people of color were systematically kept down, and what they could do to resist. The women drew from and looked beyond personal experiences to examine societal problems of control and domination and to explore possibilities for social change. They talked about going together to a candlelight vigil protesting violence against women, which had been organized for the following week. Some of the women had never been involved in a political action before. When the facilitator had first told them about this vigil, only Diane had expressed interest in going, but by the end of the group meeting the group members had all resolved to go together, and several said they would bring their friends. The group was highly energized when it came to a close. The idea of doing something active "outside" that had shared meaning to them "inside" was exciting. As Lori summed it up: "I may sound off a lot in the group, but I feel really helpless when it comes to actually changing things. I know I can't do much to make an impact all by myself, but I think if we work together we can really make a difference."

This group example reflects the integration of personal and political content in groups that emphasize consciousness-raising, support, and social action. Small groups such as this one built alliances with other groups as they fought to combat patriarchal relationships at the personal, interpersonal, and societal levels. It was seen as important that empowerment-oriented groups examined the internal diversity of the group in order to celebrate it and keep it from being a divisive force. The worker's ability to move with the group in a non-directive but active fashion, facilitating a discussion of intimate personal issues one moment, and helping the group reflect on broader social implications the next, was key to successful feminist group work.

A psychiatric survivors' group

This second group example has some elements similar to the first, particularly its non-elitist approach to group facilitation and its efforts to make connections between personal and political concerns. It differs in being a mixed-sex group and less focused on social action goals. The group was formed at a recipient-directed mental health organization with historic ties to the mental patients' liberation movement (Chamberlin 1990). The organization was structured as a social club, and was committed to consciously avoiding the negative labeling of its members, emphasizing members' rights, promoting an awareness of power relationships within the mental health system, and actively opposing oppression. The psychiatric survivors' group was developed and facilitated by a female social work student, at the request of several of those who became its members. It was a group for service recipients who wanted to explore their experiences as survivors of the mental health system and their efforts to move forward in their lives. Group meetings focused on problem solving and peer support around personal and interpersonal issues such as relationship difficulties, family problems, and issues related to coping with disabilities and the pervasiveness of societal stigma and prejudice.

This was an open membership mixed-gender group, with a core group of five regulars, three women and two men. The impact of gender on group dynamics was a constant undercurrent, affecting group dynamics in several ways. Gender differences were most pronounced in the communication patterns of the group. The male members tended to dominate group discussion and to direct most of their comments towards the facilitator, while the women interacted more with each other, functioning as an internal mutual-aid sub-group. Concerns about sexism periodically emerged, interacting with awareness of discrimination against users of psychiatric services, as in the meeting described below. In this session, a heated discussion ensued when Dennis, a man in his thirties who had been in the mental health system since adolescence, made an announcement:

Dennis: I decided to quit coming here. (*Turning to the facilitator*) I have to get out of the place if I am ever going to start meeting girls. I'm going to quit coming here, Steffi.

Steffi (the student facilitating the group): Wow, Dennis, that's quite a big decision. Why don't you tell the group, instead of me.

Dennis: Well, no offence to you guys, I really like all of you. I like coming here to the club, but I want to live a normal life, with normal friends and especially girlfriends. I don't want people to know about my mental illness and I don't want to date girls who are mentally ill.

Kate (late thirties, very active in the disability rights movement): Dennis, that insults all of us! Are you ashamed of who you are?

Dennis: Well, no, not ashamed but. . . . I meet girls, pretty girls, and I ask them out, but when they find out I've been in the hospital, or that I come here, all of a sudden they are not interested.

Gloria (mid-fifties, a member of the organization for almost twenty years): Well, there are plenty of women here who like you, Dennis. I don't know why you are so hung up on being so-called "normal." You have so many friends here, do you really want to cut yourself off from them?

Cheri (in her early thirties, recently discharged from a local psychiatric facility): I have felt so much better about myself since coming here, people don't call you crazy here and put you down. I come almost every day. I can't imagine wanting to leave.

Jimmy (a relatively new member, in his twenties; *to Steffi*): I like the girls here just fine (*winking*). I don't see all that much difference between the girls here and girls who are not mentally ill.

Kate: That's the whole point, Jimmy, there are no real differences, just different experiences—

Jimmy (*interrupting Kate*): The girls I have dated who have never been in the hospital are just as crazy as anyone else.

Kate: Yes, as I was saying before you interrupted me, the differences are that most of us have had some pretty awful experiences: we have experienced repeated trauma, have been abused by our families and by the mental health system.

You want so badly to have girls think you are normal, but you have been through a lot in your life. Are you ready to just deny it? You are implying that we are not good enough for you, and that you are not good enough.

Gloria: This sounds like what we were talking about last week, about internalized oppression.

Steffi: I think you are right, Gloria. Can you say more about that?

Gloria: Dennis, I think you are reacting to the stigma against people who are mentally ill by internalizing it, identifying with the prejudice, saying mentally ill girls aren't as good as girls who aren't mentally ill. It's self-hate—

Dennis: That's not true.

Steffi: Dennis, please let Gloria finish what she's saying.

Gloria: I also think what he is saying is sexist, like talking about whether the girls are pretty, and making such a big deal of it.

Steffi: So, maybe we are talking about several different kinds of oppression.

As the discussion progressed, the focus shifted away from Dennis's announcement to the prejudice – and the self-hate – many of the members had experienced and how they had attempted to cope with them. Dennis denied that he had been sexist in his earlier remarks but was able to hear other group members explain how different forms of oppression can be similar, how they can feed off each other, reinforcing the notion that some people are inferior and second rate.

Conclusion

These two group practice examples are offered as glimpses into what gendered analysis can do to deepen our understanding of group principles and processes and to ensure that both women and men benefit from the group experience. To what extent does a gendered approach based on social action goals and feminist principles have anything to offer to women and to men in contemporary practice? That will be explored in subsequent chapters. Also emphasized throughout the rest of the book is the diversity within the category "women," both in relation to specific groupings of women (a range of disabled women, of older women, of women with health problems, for instance) meeting together in particular settings, and also in relation to the overlaps and interactions between these various groupings.

The other postmodernist challenges to women organizing together in feminist social action groups – the rethinking of power and the refutation of dichotomy between male and female, for example – will also recur throughout this book. Whether they result in a weakening of the sense of shared goals for change characteristic of the heady days of anti-oppressive social action is for the reader to judge. It is already clear though, that Foucauldian concepts of resistance (Foucault 1979; Sheridan 1980) are nothing new in group work.

References

Breton, M. (1995) "The potential for social action in groups," *Social Work With Groups*, 18, 2–3: 5–13.

Bricker-Jenkins, M., Hooyman, N.R. and Gottlieb, N. (eds) (1991) *Feminist Social Work Practice in Clinical Settings*, Newbury Park, CA: Sage Publications.

Butler, S. and Wintram, C. (1991) *Feminist Groupwork*, London: Sage Publications.

Chamberlin, J. (1990) "The ex-patients movement: here we've been and where we're going," *Journal of Mind and Behavior*, 11, 3–4: 323–36.

Cohen, M.B. (1994) "'Who wants to chair the meeting?' Group development and leadership patterns in a community action group of homeless people," *Social Work With Groups*, 17, 1–2: 81–7.

Cohen, M.B. and Mullender, A. (1999) "The personal in the political: exploring the group work continuum from individual to social change goals," *Social Work With Groups*, 22, 1: 13–31.

Foucault, M. (1979) *The History of Sexuality, Volume 1: An Introduction*, trans. Robert Hurley, London: Allen Lane.

Freeman, J. (1972–3) "The tyranny of structurelessness," *Berkeley Journal of Sociology*, xvii: 151–64.

Gutiérrez, L.M. (1991) "Empowering women of color: a feminist approach", in Bricker-Jenkins, M., Hoyman, N. and Gottleib, N., (eds) *Feminist Social Work Practice in Clinical Settings*, Newbury Park, CA: Sage Publications.

Gutiérrez, L.M. and Lewis, E.A. (1999) *Empowering Women of Color*, New York: Columbia University Press.

Jordan, J.V., Kaplan, A.G., Miller, J.B., Stiver, I.P., and Surrey, J.L. (eds) (1991) *Women's Growth in Connection: Writings from the Stone Center*, New York: Guilford Press.

Lee, J.A.B. (1994) *The Empowerment Approach to Social Work Practice*, New York: Columbia.

Mullender, A. and Ward, D. (1991) *Self-Directed Groupwork: Users Take Action for Empowerment*, London: Whiting & Birch.

Papell, C. and Rothman, B. (1966) "Social group work models: possession and heritage," *Journal of Education for Social Work*, 2: 66–77.

Saulnier, C.F. (2000) "Incorporating feminist theory into social work practice," *Social Work With Groups*, 23, 1: 5–29.

Sheridan, A. (1980) *Michael Foucault: The Will to Truth*, London: Tavistock.

Chapter 4

Difference, collective action and women's groups

South Asian women in Britain

Ravi K. Thiara

Introduction

Given the wider racialization and gendering of British society, the dis/location of South Asian[1] women in postwar Britain is determined by the intersections of race, ethnicity, gender and class. Historically, South Asian women have been at the forefront of organizing against their oppressions, thereby challenging dominant constructions of themselves as racialized and gendered objects. The formation of autonomous feminist groups and networks has been a feature of South Asian women's activism since the 1970s, resulting in a challenge to earlier invisibilities and representations of black[2] women, itself a part of a bigger project of deconstruction initiated by black feminists in the 1970s. In recent years, poststructuralism and postmodernism have created a theoretical space for discourse about difference, subjectivity and agency, allowing black women to be foregrounded and the notion of 'blackness' itself to be interrogated. The implications and impact of this on action, however, have been greatly debated. What have discourses of 'difference' meant for South Asian women and collective action? What have been the commonalities and differences among South Asian women? Indeed, has the 'common' been sufficient to enable collective action? How have recent developments in community action impacted on women's action? How has action through the formation of women's groups facilitated personal–social transformation and generated a collective awareness and politicization for such women? These are some of the questions examined in this chapter in relation to the history of collective action by South Asian women, by locating it within the broader frame of anti-racist struggles since the 1970s, while an example of a women's group in the Midlands will be used to further explore how some of these issues have operated at a practical level. The chapter seeks to demonstrate the multiple, complex and contradictory locations of South Asian women in resistance politics in Britain and the ways in which they have sought to use women's groups to construct and articulate women's interests and issues.

South Asian women and collective action

At the outset, it has to be emphasized that the term 'Asian', itself constructed in Britain, encompasses diverse groups with differing histories, interests and experiences.[3] Given this complexity, it is necessary to further deconstruct the category 'South Asian women' as it encompasses a highly heterogeneous group marked by differences of geographical origin, language, class, religion and caste. As insightfully discussed by Brah (1992: 64), the accompanying cultural and gender systems are equally different. Although similarity in their structural location results in much commonality, the particular history of migration has led to differing issues and concerns for the different categories of South Asian women.[4] So, for Sikh women, who were among the earlier migrants, key issues relate to redundancies and unemployment at a time of radical change in the nature of employment, while for Bangladeshi women, who migrated later, exclusion from the labour market has been an issue along with inadequate housing and racist attacks. Thus to speak of the 'real' or 'authentic' South Asian homogenizes/naturalizes this category, making it important to problematize the notion of a unitary South Asian woman's experience by highlighting the complex and multidimensional nature of their knowledges, experiences and narratives. In underlining this understanding, this chapter looks at the ways in which South Asian women have attempted to challenge racialized exclusions as well as to transform social relations within families and communities as gendered subjects.

Community action,[5] albeit of changing kinds, has been the principle arena through which minority communities in Britain have sought to assert their sense of belonging and to challenge dominant constructions.[6] Questions of identity and subjectivity have been central to both black community politics and black women's action in 1970s and 1980s Britain. Writers have increasingly argued for subjectivity to be viewed as dynamic, multiple and socially and historically produced, often involving contradictory experiential situations and changing social, cultural and political conditions (Mama 1995: 159). In relation to South Asian women, gendered and racialized social relations, in articulation with state policies and discursive practices, have impacted on the formation of their subjectivity. State racism in Britain targeted at South Asian groups has been historically legitimized through a particular ideological construction of Asian marriage and family systems (Brah 1992: 68). Much of the contemporary popular, academic and political discourse continues to represent South Asian women as the passive victims of out-of-date male-dominated traditions and practices, as witnessed in recurrent press reports of arranged marriages,[7] which have often been the only visibility accorded to South Asian women. Deprived of their agency/subjectivity, women are depicted as the 'done to' rather than the 'doers', and outmoded cultural practices are seen as the culprits. Furthermore, Asian culture is presented as an unchanging essence instead of being understood as a continuously constitutive and contested dynamic that also presents a possible site of resistance for minority communities. Indeed, South Asian women's organizations have constantly emphasized the need for Asian women to make their own choices about how and why they challenge their marriage systems within a context where Asian marriages have become so deeply ingrained within racialized discourses (Trivedi 1984). While an important site of tension, negotiation and challenge, the issue of marriage is not the only significant factor for South Asian women, as amply demonstrated by the challenges they have posed both at discursive and practical levels over the last three decades.

Both anti-racist struggles and the development of the black feminist movement provide important backdrops for an understanding of collective action by South Asian women. This movement, an organic development in the 1970s during a period of heightened racism, was grounded in the everyday material reality and struggles of black women against both societal racism and the challenges posed to women by their disempowering location within their own communities. While some parallels existed with the white women's liberation movement (WLM), the latter was also critiqued for its failure to take on the specificity of black women in its universalizing claims. Thus autonomous black women's organizations resulted both from the lack of attention being given to the particularity of black women within feminist theory and practice and from the marginalizing of gender issues within black organizations. The birth of feminist black women's groups and networks introduced a new dimension into the political agenda.

Critiquing both feminist theory and white feminist agendas, black feminism emphasized the international context of race, class and imperialism, and demanded that primacy not be given to one but that the intersections of all be examined. Black feminists such as Hazel Carby stressed the need to take account of the global social relations of power and the ways in which Western feminism served to reproduce the categories through which the 'West' constructs itself as superior to 'others' (Carby 1982). Additionally, some of the central categories of feminism were critiqued, along with the invisibility and representation of the 'other' in feminist discourse (see *Feminist Review* 1984, 17). Emphasis on 'difference' was the main way through which racism in feminist theory and practice was challenged and exposed so that, by the 1990s, 'woman' as a unitary category no longer had currency either among activists or within feminist theory (see also Hill-Collins 1991).

At a practical level, though localized contexts determined priorities, black women's groups aimed to challenge the specific oppression resulting from the intersections of racism, sexism and class faced by different categories of black women. Early organizations faced the contradiction of forming broad-based alliances while asserting distinctiveness and specificity. Attempts to retain sensitivity to difference among black women while developing effective political strategies revealed numerous tensions between women on various political issues. These ranged from differences in the analysis of racism *vis-à-vis* other systems of inequality through to those between feminists and non-feminists, all resulting in different priorities and strategies (Brah 1992: 10). Identity politics and an emphasis on authenticity of personal experience also led to some women building hierarchies of oppression that were less helpful.

This wider context and the diverse manifestation and evolution of collective action by South Asian women, reflected in a range of political opinions and projects, makes the task of categorizing such organizations a difficult one. What is worthy of note is that resistance by South Asian women has deep historical roots both in the subcontinent and in Britain. Whether through feminist collectives or in religious and welfare groups, the central aim of South Asian women has been to create supportive and enabling contexts for women who have a broadly shared experience. Activities have generally centred around the need to: provide appropriate information, support and advice; challenge injustice and racist practices through campaigning work; organize social and cultural activities; and provide education and training, as well as space for women to organize politically around issues defined as relevant to their lives. Irrespective of their own political leanings, groups have also built alliances with other organizations in order to make a statement about their dis/location in British society.

Phizacklea and Miles (1987) and Brah (1992), among others, highlight the range of South Asian women's action – ranging from industrial disputes, immigration and defence campaigns, to public protests against racist harassment and violence against women. Historically, immigration has been one of the major areas for Asian women's organizations. State-orchestrated witch-hunts against 'arranged marriages' have served to victimize women and, through the enforcing of the primary purpose rule,[8] humiliating 'virginity tests' and X-ray examinations,[9] have frustrated their attempts to establish normal family life in Britain. As a response to racist and sexist immigration practices, numerous anti-deportation campaigns have been spearheaded and successfully fought by Asian women's organizations (see Trivedi 1994: 45–6). The issue of violence against women has also been key for women's groups, resulting in the establishing of Asian women's refuge (shelter) support services throughout the country. These have challenged racism within the refuge movement as well as the largely male assumption that violence is not a problem within their own communities. Committed organization by South Asian women has served to raise the public profile of the issue of men's violence, achieved through a combination of public demonstrations and the setting up of services, conferences and campaigns. Southall Black Sisters' support for Kiranjeet Ahluwalia[10] (a woman imprisoned for the murder of her abusive husband and later released after concerted campaigning) clearly captured the public attention and is one aspect of the range of continuing protest action by South Asian women in Britain.

This dynamic history of collective action, seeking to build unity not only across 'race' but ethnicity, religion, caste and regional differences, throws up many questions. To what extent have South Asian women's organizations attempted to establish distinctive (ethnic) cultural and political institutions in their bid to establish autonomy? Or should they be seen as an implicit rejection of the 'communal option' and an attempt to build broader agendas based on commonality of experience in their objective of self-determination, control and recognition? As noted, much of the mobilization by South Asian women has been around the issue of violence against women. This has challenged both their gendered and their racialized identities, involving many contradictions and tensions as it has become not only an arena for women to expose Western orientalist constructions of them as 'passive' and 'exotic' objects but also a vehicle for challenging those practices that are detrimental to women. It is a challenge that continues, as South Asian women try to define and foreground their subjectivity as a complex and multiple reality. For many individuals, South Asian women's organizations have been a source of nurture and development, especially for those women who sought a political home; the fact that such organizations have also constituted a platform for the building of individual careers is not to be overlooked. Critical debate about the extent to which the leadership of women's groups has managed to reflect their wider constituencies continues even today, but the involvement of numerous 'ordinary' women in many key struggles is testimony to the attempts many groups have made to ensure that they do not become divorced from those whom they seek to represent.

The issue of funding has been crucial in the development, survival and agenda setting of most community organizations and is an important issue for South Asian women. According to Werbner and Anwar, 'state funding also depends on "fictions" of communal unity; it both divides immigrant communities . . . into discrete ethnic groups, and implies that each such group is an undivided unity . . .' (Werbner and Anwar 1991: 33). While recognizing the positive role of state funding – in the regularizing of procedures and accountability structures and the appointment of professionals – many activists and writers have argued that professionalization has led to a depoliticizing and bureaucratizing of collective action and 'community' protest politics. The demand for autonomy on the one hand and the right to state funds (dependence) on the other has produced critical quandaries for South Asian women's organizations. Negotiation, reform and protest have tended to mark the numerous local and national struggles waged by such groups. Generally, there has been a shift from direct action against the state to intra-ethnic competition over scant resources, leading to fragmentation and a reduced potential for solidarity. Thus radicalism has often been reduced to the level of rhetoric and the reality has been determined by negotiation and accommodation in contexts where it is difficult for groups to set their own agendas (Eade 1989). Indeed, more generally, there has been a dramatic change in black resistance politics during the 1980s and 1990s, a period marked by greater fragmentation and competition for state-allocated resources between minority communities and groups.

An example

As already noted, male violence has been a key issue around which South Asian women have organized throughout the major cities of Britain since the late 1970s. Having outlined some of the main issues in relation to collective action by South Asian women, I now turn to a discussion of a women's group set up in the East Midlands in the latter part of the 1980s in order to explore these issues a little further. The group, comprised of women from diverse professional (social work, probation, welfare rights, education, housing) and religious/ethnic (Hindu, Muslim, Sikh) backgrounds, began informally to discuss in their various work settings issues of male and family violence that individuals were increasingly encountering. These incidents and the often inappropriate responses that South Asian women were experiencing both within refuge support services and from other white professionals led this informal grouping to consider ways in which specialized services could be set up while also challenging existing practice.

Initial discussions were marked both by a condemnation of male violence within their communities (cases were known to some group members), anger at the way in which male leaders sought to deny its existence, and a careful consideration of the implications of challenging such practices within a racialized context. Women made the decision to name unacceptable practices within South Asian communities as well as the wider racism in society. In particular, the group was sensitive to the male construction of them as 'family breakers' or 'Westernized women' who had nothing in common with women in their communities, while, on the other hand, they sought to challenge the stereotype of the oppressed Asian woman. In practice, this often meant being extremely aware of their actions such as the use of 'dress' to make a statement – for example, wearing *salwar kameez* (traditional tunic and trousers) to address council meetings attended by both Asian leaders and white politicians. One woman recounts how a white male politician had been greatly surprised at her 'articulate speech' when he had expected her to be barely able to speak English, based on the fact that she was traditionally dressed. The group spent much time deliberating on the strategies that would be adopted in different settings to make political statements about South Asian women in Britain.

Obstruction by male community leaders was a major issue for the group, especially as it often went hand in hand with a cultural relativism practised by white professionals (see below). The group consisted both of women who were from local communities and of those who had moved from other geographical areas, leading to different experiences of male obstruction and community response. For those who lived in their communities the risk was the greatest, with a regular trickle of people wanting to get information on women who were being assisted by the group. This included giving a 'bad name' to, and other reprisals against, individuals who came to be known for helping these women, leading some activists to withhold their involvement even from their families. One of the ways this was tackled, as a project became operational for South Asian women, was to recruit workers from outside the area to lessen the potential risk. This issue was regularly addressed at meetings, and strategies were worked out to minimize danger as well as for hearing individual concerns. At times, individual women adopted a lower profile in the group to lessen the risk to themselves.

The fact that many of the women were professionals in their own right created some space for them to challenge the cultural relativism in the practice of white professionals. One of the key recurrent issues was the 'hands-off' approach adopted by many in respect of South Asian women, which resulted in collusion with male leaders on the one hand and inappropriate actions on the other. As has been highlighted by Hanana Siddiqui of Southall Black Sisters, the acceptance of men as spokespersons for their communities and non-interference on the part of professionals are major issues for South Asian women's groups even today:

> those outside these communities feel that they can't interfere, that they have to tolerate other cultures and that to interfere might even be racist. . . . We have to battle to get women's voices heard. Our wishes, our demands and our interests are not represented by community leaders who tend to be the most conservative, patriarchal and religious forces in the community . . . we demand something different: we do want intervention but it has to be sensitive.
>
> (Quoted in Griffin 1995)

The diversity that marked the backgrounds of group members – of religion, caste, ethnicity, class and region – coincided with those of service users. Accommodating difference meant giving careful attention to the planning of services in the refuge – different kitchens to accommodate Muslim, Sikh and Hindu women as well as leisure materials and other resources that were culturally appropriate. At the same time, the group sought to organize around issues that were common to women across different cultural and ethnic groups; this often went against the grain of male-dominated community politics which increasingly reinforced cultural differences. Consequently, women in the group were seen by 'community leaders' as damaging the interests of the ethnic group since they engaged in an internal critique, the men taking a view that equates action with group benefits rather than that which also contests and attempts to transform inequalities within as well as without. This is an experience common to many feminist South Asian women's groups whose members have sought to provide a critique in action of the formulations of 'community'. Some of the questions constantly raised by women are 'which community, whose view of the community, and who benefits in the community?', pointing out that male leaders have tended to construct the concept for their own benefits. Yet, when carrying out consultation with the community, welfare agencies have gone to such leaders and overlooked the voices and views of women. Issues of 'community' and 'empowerment' are powerfully critiqued in the writing of Yuval-Davis, who stresses the need to problematize such notions:

> [T]he 'naturalness' of the 'community' assumes a given collectivity with given boundaries – it allows for internal growth and probably differentiation but not for ideological and material reconstructions of the boundaries themselves. It does not allow for collectivities to be seen as social constructs whose boundaries, structures and norms are the result of constant processes of struggles and negotiations or more general social developments.
>
> (1994: 181)

Just as the existence of black people exposed dominant formulations of the 'English community' as racist and exclusive, many South Asian women's organizations posed a challenge to the notion of the wholeness of a 'community' with 'leaders', seeing this as a chauvinistically constructed collectivity. Similarly, the existence of conflicting interests (as between men and women, young and old, Asian and African-Caribbean) is overlooked by discourses on empowerment which include an 'automatic assumption of a progressive connotation of the "empowerment of the people", assuming a non-problematic transition from individual to collective power, as well as a pre-given, non-problematic definition of the boundaries of "the people"' (Yuval-Davis 1994: 181).

It is apparent from the history of community action in Britain that the construction of 'difference' has depended on the purpose and outcomes of such action, hence the same categories of people have been constructed differently for various political projects (e.g. 'Paki' by the extreme right-wing, 'black British' by those seeking to unite across difference against racism, and more recently 'Muslim fundamentalist' by those engaged in anti-Islamic discourse). For instance, South Asian women's organizations often developed new boundaries and included those previously defined as outsiders so that 'Asian' encompassed Sikh, Muslim and Hindu, as in the example above. This was pertinent only within the context of Britain, where racism was a common concern, since relations between the three religious groups in the subcontinent are marked by deep political mistrust and exclusivist constructions of the nation state. Even in the British context, there has been a shift towards a narrowing of identities, shaped in part by increasingly divergent dis/locations and in part by discourses around 'Muslims'.[11] All of this poses important questions about action by women's groups. Should differences be overlooked in the interests of the group? Are group solidarity and collective action always desirable? Under what conditions does the ideal of an overarching commonality become unacceptable or untenable?

These questions were constantly faced by the women's group in question, which challenged the notion of 'community leaders' but also had to face the fact that most of its membership was drawn from educated professional women. While attempts were made to incorporate 'ordinary women' into the group through the involve-ment of survivors of violence, this remained an unresolved issue. The group was agreed, however, in reinforcing the view that it was not representative of all South Asian women but acted more as an advocate for some of their issues. While the group was focused around issues affecting South Asian women, most of the members had a political commitment to a common black struggle – at a time when the term 'black' was becoming contested (see next section). It was recognized that individuals would construct their identity in changing ways and locate them-selves in more than one group at any one time. The need to preserve and construct positive collective and personal identities within a racialized context was constantly recognized – decisions were made to have an anti-racist stance, in common with other black groups, but to leave space for individuals to have their own definitions. Carving out these positive identities resulted in certain costs and contradictions and members were often accused of divisiveness when emphasizing their specificity.

'Difference' and action

As discussed in the introductory chapter to this book and illustrated by the example of the group in this chapter, poststructuralist and postmodernist discourses have warned against homogeneous categories, thus undermining the notion of a unitary racism. Indeed, the contemporary period is marked by the emergence of 'new ethnicities' and a complexity of racisms, on the one hand, and a fragmentation of 'blackness' as a political identity, with a foregrounding of ethnic and cultural difference, on the other (Hall 1988; Solomos and Back 1995). Much of the debate within black organizations and politics has focused on the issue of 'black' and its applicability as an overarching political identity for both African-Caribbean and South Asian groups. While black groups migrating to Britain were differentially racialized, their structural location within major areas of life created some commonalities around the processes of racism. Influenced by the Black Power movement in the USA, where 'black' became a label of pride, the term was increasingly used by both South Asian and African-Caribbean organizations and activists in the 1970s in an attempt to foster solidarity. However, debate about the applicability of 'black' has been extensive since the late 1980s, first articulated by Hazareesingh (1986) and Modood (1988), and amply aired elsewhere (see Brah 1992). What this argument sought to do was emphasize cultural difference at the expense of a politics of unity against racism; in the process it failed, some argued, to recognize that political and cultural meanings could differ across contexts. Moreover, the primacy given to cultural difference was seen as 'ethnicism' by critics like Brah, who argued that 'it posits "ethnic difference" as the primary modality around which social life is constituted and experienced' (1996: 99), thus defining cultural needs in isolation from experiences that are textured by racism, class or gender. This led to an inherent implication that a culturally different group is somehow internally homogenous. This debate has been important in highlighting the diverse cultures among South Asian groups, which in themselves are under-pinned by caste, class, religious, regional and linguistic differences. There is an increasing recognition that, while poststructuralism has created a space for theorizing about 'difference', such theories have not always translated into practical organization.

As already noted, in the 1990s this critique was reflected in the development towards the ethnicizing, professionalizing and depoliticizing of community politics, resulting often in a greater emphasis on 'acceptable' and 'safe' issues. The concept 'black' came to be replaced by other markers of difference, such as 'Asian/Muslim/Indian'; labels that sought to mobilize different cultural, religious and political identities for differing political purposes and outcomes. At the same time, descriptors such as 'black' were increasingly stripped of their political use and used to refer only to people of African-Caribbean origin, clearly illustrated by the adoption of this category in this way in the 1991 Census, for instance. Thus it has become confusing to use 'black' as an overarching category, with the term 'black and minority ethnic' now having greater currency.

Given that poststructuralism has proffered new ways of addressing complex social realities, it is also important in its insights for feminist thought and practice, including in groups. Indeed, as noted earlier, discussions of difference have become central. While the role of 'race' in creating racialized categories is recognized, the need to avoid a reinforcing of essentialist notions of difference (i.e. the idea that there exists a pure essence across cultural and historical barriers) is emphasized. Thus, while earlier black feminist discourse stressed the specificity of black women, recently we have been urged to guard against essentializing this specificity, so that 'black and white feminism should not be seen as essentially fixed oppositional categories but rather as historically contingent fields of contestation within discursive and material practices' (Brah 1992: 1).

Given the poststructuralist foregrounding of difference, the issue facing feminism concerns the extent to which such a discursive position empowers and enables collective political action at a concrete level. How can the emphasis on difference constructively inform and feed into a material politics that is founded on contradictions and conflicts? How can commonalities be built across axes of difference? Some writers, Yuval-Davis for instance, have bravely argued for a 'coalition politics' view, where the 'differences among women are recognized and given a voice, without fixating the boundaries of this coalition in terms of "who" we are but in terms of what we want to achieve' (1994: 189). Although her 'transversal politics' framework is useful,[12] it overlooks both the fact that coalitions can be built across those differences that are more acceptable, powerful and privileged, and the existence of differences that are not always reconcilable. It potentially reduces, too, the broader goal of transforming social relations to smaller issue-based struggles and gains. Brah argues that, when talking about difference, it is important to ask whether difference affirms diversity or is used for discriminatory and exclusionary practices. She stresses the need to address the issue of how different groups of women are represented and how women construct and represent their specific experiences, as well as the circumstances under which difference is used to assert a collective identity (Brah 1992).

Conclusion

This chapter has sought to highlight how racialized identities located within gendered social relations pose complex problems for women seeking to challenge and transform social relations. Collective action by South Asian women, marked by tension and contradiction, has challenged both masculinist 'community' politics and racist discursive and material practices in postwar Britain. Through a range of strategies, including political and cultural activism, consciousness-raising and interpersonal relationships, South Asian women have sought to cope with and confront this dominant order. The example of a particular South Asian women's group has illustrated how 'difference' can be both recognized and encompassed in organizing services to respond to women's wider needs that result from male violence and abuse, while bearing in mind the context of the wider community and society.

The complex reality of South Asian women who are themselves active at a number of levels has been underlined to demonstrate how their multidimensionality has challenged existing discourse. While warning against promoting an essentialist notion of South Asian women and of Asian communities, it has been argued that much of the existing discourse retains 'community' as a universalizing and homogenizing category that subsumes class, gender, age, generation and spatial differences. Moreover, the notion of identity as multiple, complex and situational has been emphasized, together with the need to deconstruct the uncritically accepted notion of 'community leaders and representatives'.

Notes

1 'South Asian' refers to people whose origins lie in India, Pakistan, Bangladesh and Sri Lanka. The terms 'South Asian' and 'Asian' are sometimes used interchangeably.

2 Where I use the term 'black' it refers collectively to all minority groups who are subjected to anti-black racism. (See also p. 49.)

3 South Asian migration to Britain was part of the larger postwar migration flow when black labour was recruited to meet widespread labour shortages. This has been insightfully documented by a number of scholars (see Layton-Henry 1984; Anwar 1986; Solomos 1989).

4 Within the migration flow, Indian women arrived in Britain before those from Pakistan and Bangladesh, and were drawn into the labour market, often in low-paid unskilled and semi-skilled work, or as homeworkers. Today, South Asian women are mainly concentrated in the West Midlands, Greater London and West Yorkshire; Indian women constitute the largest group in Greater London and the West Midlands whereas Pakistani women predominate in West Yorkshire, while the largest percentage of Bangladeshi women is to be found in Greater London (Owen 1994: 34).

5 Although there is an increasing body of literature on 'ethnic mobilization', much of the writing has tended either to remain silent about or to marginalize the struggles that South Asian women have forged through autonomous groups and networks.

6 It has been estimated that, at the beginning of the 1990s, there were approximately 2,000 minority ethnic organizations (Werbner and Anwar 1991: 13).

7 Recent government and activist attention to 'forced marriages', especially the campaigning by Southall Black Sisters (1990), needs to be distinguished from the recurrent discourse around arranged marriages. Concern about young women being taken under duress by their families to be married overseas has led activists to work with the Foreign Office and the police to inform and protect young women.

8 The primary purpose rule sought to prove that a marriage was genuine and not engaged for the purpose of obtaining citizenship in the UK.

9 Groups such as Southall Black Sisters (1990) have committedly campaigned around this and similar issues, and more recently have made some important gains, especially around the primary purpose rule.

10 Kiranjeet's story is documented in *The Circle of Light* (Ahluwalia and Gupta 1997).

11 Social unrest in northern English cities in the summer of 2001, involving primarily Muslim young people, has led many non-Muslim Asian 'community leaders' and commentators to distance themselves from Muslim communities. This has been further reinforced since the events of 11 September 2001 in the USA.

12 'In "transversal politics", perceived unity and homogeneity is replaced by dialogues which give recognition to the specific positionings of those who participate in them as well as the "unfinished knowledge" that each such situated positioning can offer' (Yuval-Davis 1994: 194).

References

Ahluwalia, K. and Gupta, R. (1997) *Circle of Light: The Autobiography of Kiranjeet Ahluwalia*, London: HarperCollins.

Anwar, M. (1986) *Race and Politics*, London: Tavistock.

Brah, A. (1992) 'Difference, diversity, differentiation', in Donald, J. and Rattansi, A. (eds) *'Race', Culture and Difference*, London: Sage.

—— (1996) *Cartographies of Diaspora: Contesting Identities*, London: Routledge.

Carby, H. (1982) 'White woman listen! Black feminism and the boundaries of sisterhood', in Centre for Contemporary Cultural Studies, *The Empire Strikes Back*, London: Hutchinson.

Eade, J. (1989) *The Politics of Community: The Bangladeshi Community in East London*, Aldershot: Gower.

Feminist Review (1984) Special issue: 'Many Voices, One Chant: Black Feminist Perspectives', Autumn, 17. (Whole issue.)

Griffin, G. (1995) 'The Struggles continue – an interview with Hanana Siddiqui of Southall Black Sisters', in Griffin, G. (ed.) *Feminist Activism in the 1990s*, London: Taylor & Francis.

Hall, S. (1988) 'New ethnicities', in Mercer, K. (ed.) *Black Film, British Cinema*, ICA Document No. 7, London: British Film Institute.

Hazareesingh, S. (1986) 'Racism and cultural identity: an Indian perspective', *Dragon's Teeth*, 24: 4–10.

Hill-Collins, P. (1991) *Black Feminist Thought*, London: Routledge.

Layton-Henry, Z. (1984) *The Politics of Race in Britain*, London: Allen & Unwin.

Mama, A. (1995) *Beyond Masks: Race, Gender and Subjectivity*, London: Routledge.

Modood, T. (1988) '"Black" racial equality and Asian identity', *New Community*, XIV, 3: 397–404.

Owen, D. (1994) *Ethnic Minority Women and the Labour Market: Analysis of the 1991 Census*, London: Equal Opportunities Commission.

Phizacklea, A. and Miles, R. (1987) 'The strike at Grunwick', *New Community*, IV, 3: 268–78.

Solomos, J. (1989) *Race and Racism in Contemporary Britain*, London: Macmillan.

Solomos, J. and Back, L. (1995) *Race, Politics and Social Change*, London: Routledge.

Southall Black Sisters (1990) *Against the Grain: A Celebration of Survival and Struggle*, London: SBS.

Trivedi, P. (1984) 'To deny our fullness: Asian women in the making of history', *Feminist Review*, 17: 37–50.

Werbner, P. and Anwar, M. (eds) (1991) *Black and Ethnic Leadership: The Cultural Dimensions of Political Action*, London: Routledge.

Yuval-Davis, N. (1994) 'Women, ethnicity and empowerment', in Bhavnani, K. K. and Phoenix, A. (eds) *Shifting Identities, Shifting Racisms*, London: Sage.

Chapter 5

Critical reflections on profeminist practice in men's groups

Bob Pease

Introduction

In this chapter I take a reflective journey through my experiences of working in and engaging with all-male groups in Australia. I begin by locating my experiences within the context of the current debate on the potential and limitations of men's groups and I start the personal journey with my involvement in anti-sexist consciousness-raising groups in the 1970s and 1980s, through to profeminist social action and collaborative inquiry groups in the 1990s. I also discuss my experiences in engaging groups of men in patriarchy-awareness workshops and in challenging male bonding and collusion in men's behaviour-change groups. From these experiences, I outline some of the political quandaries arising from profeminist practice with men in groups.

Profeminism for men involves a sense of responsibility for our own and other men's sexism, and a commitment to work with women to end men's violence (Douglas 1993). It acknowledges that men benefit from the oppression of women, drawing men's attention to the privileges we receive as men and the harmful effects those privileges have on women (Thorne-Finch 1992). Profeminist men also recognize that sexism has an impact on men as well as women. To oppress others, it is necessary to *suppress* oneself. Systemic male dominance deforms men, too, as evidenced in stress-related illnesses and emotional inexpressiveness. Furthermore, not all men benefit equally from the operation of the structures of domination. Issues of ethnicity, sexuality, class, disability and age significantly affect the extent to which men benefit from patriarchy.

A profeminist perspective explains dominant masculinity in structural and cultural terms. It is important to locate men's lives in the context of patriarchy, hegemonic masculinity and the social divisions between men (see, for example, Connell 1995; Hearn 1998; and Kimmel 2000). From this perspective, for men to change, we have to reconstruct masculinity in ways that acknowledge its social dimension. That means challenging gender inequality in the public arena. As men, it is important that we confront our political position. We cannot just relinquish the reality of social power. We have to develop a conscious politics aimed at creating new laws, new values and new organizational forms. It is not enough to bring 'a new man' into existence.

This theoretical approach has significant implications for rethinking groupwork with men in a context where the sparse literature on men's groups is predominantly informed by sex role theories of masculinity (see, for example, Brooks 1998; Andronico 1999; and Cowburn and Pengally 1999).

One of the major limitations of sex role theory is that it underemphasizes the economic and political power that men exercise over women. Male and female roles are seen to be equal, thus enabling men and women to engage in a common cause against sex role oppression. What is consistently missing in sex role theory is a recognition of the extent to which men's gender identities are based upon a struggle for social power. Men clearly suffer from adhering to dominant forms of masculinity. Many men are now concluding that the social and political gains of having power over women do not outweigh the physical, social and psychological health costs incurred (Newman 1997). Most men, however, approve of and support the overall system in spite of the burdens, and they simply want more benefits and less burdens (Ball 1997). There is no evidence that liberating men from the traditional male sex role will lead to men relinquishing their privilege and power. And yet that is where traditional approaches to working with men in groups are often heading.

Before examining the potential, and the limitations, of men's groups, a comment on distinctions between men's and women's groups is warranted. A number of feminist writers have identified gender-based differences in women's and men's groups (for example, see Reed 1988; Butler and Wintram 1991; and Schiller 1995, 1997). Reed (1988) has argued that men's groups are more oriented towards competition and status-related topics, and that they foster instrumental behaviours and intellectual discussion at the expense of personal sharing and closeness. These processes are contrasted with women's groups, which are said to be more focused on personal and familial topics and which are more likely to emphasize emotional intimacy. Schiller (1995, 1997) has consequently proposed that there is a differential model of developmental stages for women's groups – what she refers to as 'the relational model'. However, to dichotomize men's and women's groups as constituting separate gender cultures does not take into account the impact that structural context, group objectives and ideological leadership have on group processes. (See also Chapter 2). For example, a profeminist men's group addressing internalized domination and a feminist women's group organizing against structural oppression may not fit into the dichotomized models proposed. We have to be careful not to essentialize men's and women's experiences in group settings when we discuss gender issues in groups.

The potential and the limitations of men's groups

The claimed benefits in men's groups

Groups for men vary considerably in their origins, objectives, membership, structure and process. They occur in a diverse range of settings and locations. Thus there are many types of group for men. They include political action, consciousness-raising, discussion, education, support, counselling and psychotherapy groups (Stein 1983).

Groupwork with men is generally based on two beliefs: first that men as a group need to change their behaviours, belief systems and affective experiences; and, second, that the medium of the group is conducive to produce such change (Stein 1983). Within this context, Stein identifies nine functions that men's groups can serve. They

- allow men who wish to change themselves as men to affiliate with a group of men who have similar values;
- provide an opportunity for men to relate to other men in an interpersonal setting without women;
- serve as a means of demonstrating to men how they behave when they are with other men;
- highlight the ways in which members have related to other significant men in their lives;
- provide a setting in which to explore special topics which are frequently difficult for men to talk about;
- lead to a greater understanding of special problems for men;
- serve to alter the nature of the adult male-to-male relationships by promoting caring and friendship between men;
- provide the opportunity to learn new patterns of relating to women; and
- serve to increase the social and political awareness of men as a basis for eliminating individual and institutional sexism.

When such group processes work well for men they are seen to involve some or all of the following: learning to listen; building trust; stressing commonality of feelings and problems; analysing the social origins of problems; providing support and feedback; developing new values in the group; and taking group action (Creane 1981).

Thus there are many positive claims made for men's groups. Andronico (1999) argues that men's groups are ideal forums in which to raise issues relevant to men in the twenty-first century. He suggests that the sense of community fostered by groups leads men to feel less isolated and alone. Brooks similarly argues that because 'men learn to be men in front of other men', then it is in front of other men that they 'can unlearn some of the more unproductive lessons about manhood and relearn and reinforce some of the more positive lessons' (1998: 104). Horne *et al.* (1999) further argue that groupwork is an effective way to assist men to achieve 'mature masculine development'. The group is seen to provide 'a safe place to ask for nurturing, role modelling, initiating, mentoring and eldering' (1999: 106). Many advocates of men's groups claim that men are freer to be expressive with each other when women are not present.

Problems identified in men's groups

The psychological and therapeutic literature on men's groups, cited above, tends to ignore the dangers and the problems associated with such groups. Profeminist writers have drawn attention to a range of issues that need to be addressed in groupwork with men.

Nearly twenty-five years ago Schein (1977: 132–4) suggested that, even when there is some level of commitment to feminism, there are dangers in men's groups. These dangers include: collusion against women; misdirecting anger towards women; avoiding challenging other men's sexism; and containing the experience within the group. Funk (1993: 130) cautions us 'to be careful not to get caught in the habit of focusing on the support and on feeling good about being men'. Similarly, Rowan (1997: 222) notes that whatever their intentions, men's groups have a tendency to 'slide into some kind of warm self-congratulation'. He says that, while such groups can provide moving experiences for the men, they seem to contribute little to challenging the patriarchal arrangements between men and women.

Male bonding has been identified by a number of writers as a problematic issue in men's groups, 'as such bonding is usually predicated on the denigration of women' (Jukes 1999: 155). Even Lionel Tiger (1984: 176), who has tended to romanticize male bonding, has acknowledged that the 'particular characteristic of the male bond is its close interconnection with aggressive and possibly violent action'. In this regard, McBride (1995: 89) has argued that any therapeutic benefit accruing to men meeting in groups needs to be 'set against and indeed [to be] counter the history of male dominance, collusion and violence' experienced in such groups.

In the context of this theoretical debate on the potential and the limitations of groupwork with men, I wish to discuss my own experience of these issues in a range of different types of men's groups.

Anti-sexist men's consciousness-raising groups

My first encounter with all-male groups was in 1977 when I co-founded an anti-sexist men's consciousness-raising group. (See Pease 1988 for a more detailed account.) Anti-sexist men's groups at that time were distinguished by their stated aim of challenging men's sexism (see for example Tolson 1977 and Hornacek 1977), in contrast to men's liberation groups, which focused more on the negative aspects of masculinity for men (see, for example, Farrell 1975; Nichols 1975).

My motivation in setting up the group came out of my need to reassess my own behaviour, attitudes and experience as a man, the initial impetus arising out of intimate involvement with a feminist woman. The group had three major objectives:

- to explore the ways in which we as men felt limited by traditional masculinity;
- to become more aware of sexist attitudes in ourselves so that we could begin to overcome ways in which we oppressed the women in our lives; and

- to explore alternative ways of relating to each other as men that broke with traditional male bonding.

There was no formal leadership or group facilitator. Our meetings were initially focused around set topics on each night. We discussed issues such as housework, homosexuality, contraception, sexual experiences, pornography, rape, masculinity, love, work and money. Sometimes, we would all read something in common, but most often we would talk personally from our own experiences and perceptions.

Most of us were trying to overcome the barriers that separated us and to achieve a higher level of emotional intimacy. Relating to other men as emotional beings, especially to their pain and their distress, and offering physical comfort were new experiences for many of us. It meant directly confronting our homophobia. However, the emotional intimacy we developed also made it difficult at times to address sexist attitudes and behaviour within the group. Sometimes, supporting men's struggles meant bolstering their egos and reinforcing sexist behaviour, and this became a source of tension within the group.

One group of men wanted to focus on the ways in which they felt oppressed as men. They did not want to hear about the privileges we held as men or the social power we held over women. A second group of men came to the conclusion that men are hopeless oppressors and that very little could be done about that either personally or politically. A third group, of which I was a part, thought that there had to be another alternative, although we didn't know what it was at the time. These tensions were unresolved, and the larger group disbanded. Those of us who were trying to reconcile the personal and the political dimensions of our experience continued to meet until travel and work took us in other directions.

One of the key issues with which men's groups need to grapple is guilt. It is often said that men need to avoid feelings of guilt which may arise from a critical examination of masculinity. As Stein (1983: 155) argues: 'Criticism of the masculine role by some feminists and dissatisfactions with men expressed by individual women can lead to a personal sense of guilt on the part of some men simply because they are men.' In this context, guilt is seen as a negative experience that prevents men from examining their personal responsibility for oppressing women. However, I think that there is a positive place for guilt – as a catalyst for cutting through complacency. Guilt is often the first overt manifestation for men of their commitment to address their sexism. To regard guilt as an unmitigated negative can serve the purpose of relieving people of the responsibility of facing their complicity in the perpetration of injustice. Difficult feelings can arise when we realize that we have been complicit in things that have caused harm to others and I believe that these feelings must be faced and dealt with rather than avoided.

The men's group clarified a number of issues for me. It helped me to change some of my practices in the private sphere: in relation to housework, sexual expression, childcare, nurturance and my use of language. However, it did not help me to clarify what I would do in the public realm. How do we move from the lounge room to the streets? Is it possible for men to engage in public political action against patriarchy, or is this a contradiction in terms? Intuitively, at that time I was aware of the many limitations of men's groups, and I was unclear about their progressive political potential.

As I write now, I believe that through an exploration of the depths of our male consciousness we can begin to clarify the social dimensions of our masculinity. I believe, though, that we need to locate our experience in the context of critical theories of men's practices. It often seems that much current work with men on issues of masculinity is unaware of critical theory and of the history of men who have grappled with these issues. There seem to be lessons from the past that are still relevant to men's groups today. One such lesson is that, like any successful consciousness-raising, this work needs to be connected to progressive political practice – in this case, profeminist practice. It is that issue I consider next.

Men Against Sexual Assault: organizing men against sexual violence

During the 1980s I became involved in various attempts to construct a collective profeminist practice in the public realm. With other men, I organized public forums on issues of masculinity, produced pamphlets on rape and on violence against women in the home, and conducted anti-sexist classes for boys in schools. However, it was not until 1989 that this work became formalized in a profeminist social action group.

Men Against Sexual Assault (MASA) was formed at a public meeting in Melbourne in December 1989 (Pease 1995). The purpose of MASA was to encourage men to take responsibility for action against sexual assault through community education, public media work and anti-sexist workshops. The premiss was that, in order to prevent men's violence, we need to develop collective interventions aimed at challenging patriarchal belief systems at a cultural level. At the outset, MASA made a commitment to liaise closely with Centres Against Sexual Assault to ensure that its activities would be supportive of the work being done by women against sexual violence. It is understandable that women are going to be cautious of men working in the area of male violence. Finding ways to ensure that we are open to women's feedback is, I believe, important. As men working with men, we have a responsibility to find ways of remaining accountable to feminist women's groups to ensure that women's interests are kept in the foreground.

The primary focus of MASA is on rape awareness education for all men. This is based on the premiss that there is a relationship between the dominant model of masculine sexuality and the prevalence of sexual assault in society. We believe that if we want to reduce the extent of sexual violence we will need to challenge the aggressiveness of dominant constructions of male sexuality and create alternative ways of being men. Towards that end, MASA became involved in a range of community education and social action activities. In addition to organizing public forums on the societal factors that perpetuate sexual assault and running anti-sexist education classes for boys in schools, MASA organized men's marches against male violence and the White Ribbon Campaign to encourage men to wear white ribbons as a statement of their opposition to men's violence. We also engaged in public media work and gave talks at community organizations, workplaces and universities on men's responsibility to challenge violence against women.

One of MASA's projects was the development of patriarchy awareness workshops based on a racism awareness model. Their aim is to address the problem of patriarchy and its impact on the lives of women, children and other men. Each workshop uses small group discussions, simulation exercises and video to explore such issues as:

- men's personal journeys in relation to gender issues;
- analyses of patriarchal culture;
- men's experience of power and domination;
- alternatives to patriarchal power;
- the impact of men's domination on women;
- social and personal blocks to men's inability to listen to women; and
- visions of, obstacles to and potential for men to change.

It is the policy of MASA to pay women working with the survivors of men's violence to attend the workshops and offer their feedback. When men get together, even if it is to analyse and question patriarchy, subtle forms of male bonding may develop. Women's presence at the workshops helps us to keep the process on track, enriches the conversations and provides a model of the ways in which we, as men, can remain accountable to women.

The development of MASA was my first experience of a relatively successful attempt to create a collective public response by men to men's violence. While doing this work, it was important to avoid becoming focused only externally – on how to raise issues with 'other men out there'. It is important that we did not focus only on the most violent and blatant forms of sexism, while ignoring how such behaviour relates to the wider experiences of male dominance of which we are all a part (Tolman et al. 1986).

How does a men's group like MASA relate to groupwork theory? There are very few examples in the groupwork literature of groups for men who oppress and disempower others. Brown is one of the few writers on groupwork to refer to actual strategies for confronting sexism, racism and other forms of discrimination in groups (see Brown 1992). However, his promotion of anti-discriminatory groupwork stands alone as a separate chapter in the most recent edition of his popular textbook, and the anti-discriminatory principles he advocates are not integrated into the group process chapters throughout the rest of the book.

Social action that involves members of dominant groupings in challenging their own privilege are even less well documented. The chapters edited by Vinik and Levin (1991) on social action, advocacy and empowerment in groupwork all focus on marginalized populations as their constituencies. Mullender and Ward's self-directed groupwork model (1991) makes an important contribution to social action groupwork. However, it also tends to be primarily oriented towards working with marginalized and disempowered groupings. One contribution to working with dominant groupings comes from programmes for violent men.

Men's behaviour-change groups

In recent years, we have witnessed a dramatic increase in the development of group counselling programmes for men who are violent to women partners. As this issue is addressed elsewhere in this book, I have only a few comments to make here about my concerns in relation to these men's groups. While I have not been directly involved in running men's behaviour-change groups, I have had the opportunity to observe the dynamics of these groups from a range of vantage points. I have sat in as an observer in a number of groups. I have been a member of a critical reference group for a profeminist men's behaviour-change programme. I have supervised two PhD students on their work in these programmes. I have also been involved in forums with group facilitators, and I have consulted with women's groups about their experiences of these groups.

In Australia, as elsewhere, some programmes for men who are violent have focused on overcoming their fears of intimacy, helping them regain self-esteem, improving communication skills and anger management, and helping them to cope better with stress. Many such programmes have become too preoccupied with the psychological sources of violence and failed to take account of the utility of violent and controlling behaviour (Adams 1988). They have embodied concepts of provocation and shared responsibility, portrayed men as helpless victims, minimized responsibility and moved towards a decriminalization of men's violence.

Working with violent men in groups is a difficult area as it involves considerations of women's safety, addressing complex issues of gender and power, and finding ways for the work to remain accountable. Edleson and Tolman (1992) have noted that, while many men report positive experiences of being in such groups, negative group effects are also apparent. Men sometimes support other men's 'negative attitudes about women or implicitly or explicitly support a man's use of abusive behaviour' (1992: 56).

When men work with men in groups it is important that they recognize their kinship with their fellow men. However, the common element that exists between male workers and male clients presents a number of problems. There is a fine line between emphasizing the commonalities among men, on the one hand, and their collusion with oppressive attitudes and behaviours, on the other (Pringle 1995: 215). When Bathrick and Kaufman audio-taped group sessions with violent men for their female supervisors, the women identified ways in which the male workers did not confront assumptions of privilege and dominance (1990: 113). If we do not challenge men's abusive and sexist behaviour, we are colluding with those behaviours.

In light of these dangers, how confrontational should men be with other men? How do we invite men to examine their behaviour without increasing their resistance to change? If we confront oppressive behaviour and attitudes too strongly, we may lose the engagement of the men being confronted. However, if we do not confront sufficiently, then we may be colluding. Men should never act in a way that condones men's victimization of women or supports their demands for patriarchal entitlement (Brooks 1998: 79). At the same time, we have to connect with men's experience. The only way through this dilemma is for men to critically reflect upon their own socialization processes and engage with their own gendered subjectivity. Thus careful monitoring is required by group facilitators, who need to confront these processes as they develop. As men and women often have different perceptions as to what constitutes collusion with participants, such monitoring further demands a process of dialogue and accountability with local feminist groups.

One of the critical problems these groups face is how to 'focus on the individual man's responsibility without losing sight of broader social and political structures?' (Hearn 1998: 198). While we have to acknowledge the importance of the individual man's responsibility for his violence, how do we avoid individualism that prevents us from developing a more structural understanding of men's violence (Hearn 1998)? Profeminist men's group facilitators say that they have addressed the concerns that feminists and refuge workers have raised about men's programmes. However, Francis and Tsang (1997: 213) argue that the feminist analysis of men's violence as 'a political problem requiring structural change is reconstructed into an interpersonal problem requiring appropriate interpersonal technique'. Thus, in their view, feminist analysis and its language have been co-opted by profeminist men's counselling groups.

A paper I wrote in 1991 (reprinted in Pease 1997) on my concerns about men's behaviour-change programmes stimulated considerable debate and controversy in Australia. The paper elicited very positive responses from many women's organizations and some male facilitators, and provoked defensive reactions from a number of other male facilitators. More than ten years later, many of my concerns about the development of these programmes in the Australian context remain unaddressed. For example:

- the lack of a policy context within government for the prevention of violence against women;
- the need for programme providers to demonstrate that their programmes are safe;
- the tendency to portray these programmes as 'the solution' to the problem of men's violence;
- the lack of integration with the criminal justice system;
- the lack of accountability to women's services;
- the lack of monitoring adherence to the existing standards; and
- the tendency to exaggerate claims of effectiveness.

I believe that this form of groupwork with men requires constant monitoring to ensure that women's safety is not further jeopardized.

Doing participatory research with profeminist men

In 1992, I undertook a participatory research project with profemininst men to explore the potential for extending profeminist men's politics into a progressive social movement (see Pease 2000). I was interested in why men become profeminist and how we might analyse men's power so as to inform a profeminst men's politics. The project, which was the subject of my PhD thesis, began with questions that have been a personal challenge in my search to understand my place as a white heterosexual man who is committed to a profeminist position. What does it mean to be a profeminist man? What is the experience of endeavouring to live out a profeminist commitment? What do these experiences tell us about re-forming men's subjectivities and practices towards gender equality? The nature of my research interests, and my commitment to praxis and change, led me to develop a participatory approach to this exploration.

It is my view that questions of political strategy are best formulated collectively. Thus, to address the formulated research aims, I invited a number of self-defined profeminist men to participate in a collaborative inquiry that would take the form of an anti-patriarchal men's consciousness-raising group. This form of action research requires a group process to enable the development of a learning community which will generate a critique of the context in which the group operates (Carr and Kemmis 1983). This learning community is further transformed into a critical one that subjects its own values and practices to scrutiny. Torbett (1991: 232) has defined the product of this process as a 'practical community of inquiry', where people are 'committed to discovering propositions about the world, life, their particular organizations and themselves that they will test in their own actions with others'. Thus, such a group process of action research involves dialogue, discussion, argumentation, critical reflection and theorizing from experience.

To begin the research, I drew up a list of twenty men whom I knew personally from my involvement in profeminist politics and who I believed would identify with a profeminist stance. Because my focus was on both personal change and political strategy, I believed it was important to choose men who were in some way taking a public stance on their profeminism. The group met twenty-two times over a period of fifteen months using consciousness-raising, collective memory work and dialogues with interlocutors to tease out the tensions and conflicts in profeminist men's politics. Confronting group members with both their allies and their opponents brings out the field of struggle. Through the dialogues, the members have to answer to interpretations that differ from their own and so modify the image they previously had of those with whom they disagree. Touraine (1988) notes that this enables participants to overcome their rationalizations as actors are encouraged to look critically at their own ideologies. The dialogues that take place model the main components of the struggle and, after the meeting with the interlocutors, the group reflects upon the encounter and analyses the action. The group works because it has to resolve the tensions between its experience and its ideology, and between its own view of the situation and that of the interlocutors.

There were five meetings with the following interlocutors: three feminist women; a men's mythopoetic ritual group; the founder of a men's rights group; a radical profeminist man who believed that it is not in men's interests to change; and two activists from a gay and lesbian rights group. These dialogues with interlocutors represented a microcosm of wider debates about the limitations of and potential for a profeminist men's politics, and they clarified directions for future profeminist interventions.

Conclusion

In light of these experiences and reflections what do I now believe is the potential in developing profeminist groupwork with men? I believe that through the process of anti-patriarchal consciousness-raising, groupwork with men can clarify the social dimensions and historical shifts in masculinities. Anti-patriarchal consciousness raising in men's groups can provide a link between personal experiences and the wider social contexts of men's lives. Men can come to understand their own sexist behaviour, to develop emotional support with other men and to encourage their anti-sexism. As a result, this form of groupwork has the potential to become an important part of profeminist practice by men.

As Thorne-Finch (1992: 270) has observed: 'Men's profeminst groups provide a forum for men to challenge themselves and other group members to look at how men contribute to the oppression and exploitation of women. This task often promotes discussion about how to avoid such complicity.' It is only recently that groupwork with men has acknowledged these issues and has begun to develop a critical focus on masculinities. This critical focus needs to be alert to the dangers in men's groups that I have discussed in this chapter and these, in turn, require the development of an overt profeminist commitment in all forms of groupwork with men.

References

Adams, D. (1988) 'Treatment models for men who batter: a profeminist analysis', in Yllo, K. and Bograd, M. (eds) *Feminist Perspectives on Wife Abuse*, Newbury Park, CA: Sage.

Andronico, P. (1999) 'Introduction', in Andronico, P. (ed.) *Men in Groups: Insights, Interventions and Psychoeducational Work*, Washington: American Psychological Association.

Ball, G. (1997) 'A psychopathology of everyday masculinity', unpublished MA thesis, La Trobe University, Melbourne.

Bathrick, D. and Kaufman, G. (1990) 'Male privilege and male violence: patriarchy's root and branch', in Abbott, F. (ed.) *Men and Intimacy*, Freedom: Crossing Press.

Brooks, G. (1998) *A New Psychotherapy for Traditional Men*, San Francisco: Jossey-Bass.

Brown, A. (1992) *Groupwork*, 3rd edn, Aldershot: Arena.

Butler, S. and Wintram, C. (1991) *Feminist Groupwork*, London: Sage.

Carr, W. and Kemmis, S. (1983) *Becoming Critical: Knowing Through Action Research*, Geelong: Deakin University Press.

Connell, R.W. (1995) *Masculinities*, Sydney: Allen & Unwin.

Cowburn, M. and Pengally, H. (1999) 'Values and processes in groupwork with men', in Wild, J. (ed.) *Working with Men for Change*, London: UCL Press.

Creane, J. (1981) 'Consciousness-raising groups for men', in Lewis, R. (ed.) *Men in Difficult Times*, Engelwood Cliffs, NJ: Prentice-Hall.

Douglas, P. (1993) 'Men = violence: a profeminist perspective on dismantling the masculine equation', Paper presented at the Second National Conference on Violence, Australian Institute of Criminology, Canberra.

Edleson, J. and Tolman, R. (1992) *Intervention for Men Who Batter: An Ecological Approach*, Newbury Park, CA: Sage.

Farrell, W. (1975) *The Liberated Man*, New York: Bantam.

Francis, B. and Tsang, A. (1997) 'War of words/words of war: a dossier on men's treatment groups in Ontario', *Canadian Social Work Review*, 11, 2: 201–20.

Funk, R. (1993) *Stopping Rape: A Challenge for Men*, Philadelphia, PA: New Society Publishers.

Hearn, J. (1998) *The Violences of Men*, London: Sage.

Hornacek, C. (1977) 'Anti-sexist consciousness-raising groups', in Snodgrass, J. (ed.) *For Men Against Sexism*, New York: Times Change Press.

Horne, A., Jolliff, D. and Roth, E. (1999) 'Men mentoring men in groups', in Andronico, P. (ed.) *Men in Groups: Insights, Interventions and Psychoeducational Work*, Washington: American Psychological Association.

Jukes, A. (1999) *Men Who Batter Women*, London: Routledge.

Kimmel, M. (2000) *The Gendered Society*, New York: Oxford University Press.

McBride, J. (1995) *War, Battering and Other Sports*, New Jersey: Humanities Press.

Mullander, A. and Ward, D. (1991) *Self-Directed Groupwork*, London: Whiting & Birch.

Newman, S. (1997) 'Men's bodies, masculinities and nursing', in Turpin, M. (ed.) *The Body in Nursing*, Melbourne: Churchill Livingston.

Nichols, J. (1975) *Men's Liberation*, New York: Penguin.

Pease, B. (1988) 'Men's groups: contradictions, limitations and political potential', in S. Regan and S. O'Higgins (eds) *Social Groupwork Monograph*, Sydney: University of Sydney Press.

Pease, B. (1995) 'MASA: Men Against Sexual Assault', in Weeks, W. and Wilson, J. (eds) *Issues Facing Australian Families*, 2nd edn, Melbourne: Longman Cheshire.

Pease, B. (1997) *Men and Sexual Politics: Towards a Profeminist Practice*, Adelaide: Dulwich Centre Publications.

Pease, B. (2000) *Recreating Men: Postmodern Masculinity Politics*, London: Sage.

Pringle, K. (1995) *Men, Masculinities and Social Welfare*, London: UCL Press.

Reed, B. (1988) 'Gender issues in groups', unpublished workshop notes.

Rowan, J. (1997) *Healing the Male Psyche: Therapy as Initiation*, London: Routledge.

Schein, L. (1977) 'Dangers with men's consciousness-raising groups', in Snodgrass, J. (ed.) *For Men Against Sexism*, New York: Times Change Press.

Schiller, L. (1995) 'Stages of development of women's groups: a relational model', in Kurland, R. and Salmon, R. (eds) *Groupwork Practice in a Troubled Society*, New York: Haworth Press.

Schiller, L. (1997) 'Rethinking stages of development in women's groups: implications for practice', *Social Work With Groups*, 20, 3: 3–19.

Stein, M. (1983) 'An overview of men's groups', in Reed, B. and Garvin, C. (eds) *Groupwork with Women/Groupwork with Men: An Overview of Gender Issues in Social Groupwork Practices*, Binghamton, New York: Haworth Press.

Thorne-Finch, R. (1992) *Ending the Silence: The Origins and Treatment of Male Violence Against Women*, Toronto: University of Toronto Press.

Tiger, L. (1984) *Men in Groups*, New York: Marion Boyars.

Tolman, R., Mowry, D., Jones, L. and Brekke, J. (1986) 'Developing a profeminist commitment among men in social work', in Van Den Bergh, N. and Cooper, L. (eds) *Feminist Visions for Social Work*, New York: National Association of Social Workers.

Tolson, A. (1977) *The Limits of Masculinity*, London: Tavistock.

Torbett, W. (1991) *The Power of Balance: Transforming Self, Society and Scientific Inquiry*, Newbury Park, CA: Sage.

Touraine, A. (1988) *Return of the Actor*, Minneapolis: University of Minnesota Press.

Vinik, A. and Levin, M. (eds) (1991) *Social Action in Groupwork*, New York: Haworth Press.

Chapter 6

Gender awareness and the role of the groupworker in programmes for domestic violence perpetrators

Neil Blacklock

Specialist groupwork programmes for domestic violence perpetrators have been running in the UK since the beginning of the 1990s. Influential manuals have been produced for the UK context (Morran and Wilson 1997; Iwi and Todd 2000); scoping surveys have been undertaken (Scourfield 1994; Mullender 1996; Mullender and Burton 2001); and evaluative research has shown success rates comparable with those in other countries (Dobash *et al.* 2000). The past five years have seen an increasing convergence in the basic content and guiding principles of all UK groups, coming to fruition when Respect (2000), the National Association for Domestic Violence Perpetrator Programmes and Associated Support Services, set out minimum standards of practice. The remaining differences, apart from the extent to which the guidelines are actually observed in practice (Mullender and Burton 2001), revolve largely around whether or not a programme is working in an integrated manner with women's services and is engaged in wider systems of anti-sexist activism. In other words, the extent to which the programme has been worked through and the gender implications of this are apparent in the delivery of the programme. Beyond that, all the established projects in the UK are delivering broadly similar programmes but with their own individual styles and identity. Group leaders tend to develop materials that play to their own strengths and there is also an increasing use of creative methods to respond to differing learning styles. Some regional variations have sprung up, such as dialect terms in Scottish groupwork materials and a particularly close link there with alcohol services. All the groups signing up to Respect's principles are working from a feminist understanding of the causes of men's violence towards women (Pence and Paymar 1990, 1996).

Almost all programmes consist of a structured programme of work designed to challenge the range of abusive behaviours deployed by perpetrators of domestic violence. Most perpetrator programmes cover the following themes (Iwi and Todd 2000):

- physical and sexual violence
- emotional abuse
- isolation and jealous behaviour

- minimizing, denial and blaming
- using children
- sexual abuse
- male privilege and economic abuse
- blocking women's anger
- harassing and stalking
- threats, coercion and intimidation.

Within each of these themes, groupworkers address issues of safety, responsibility, control, beliefs, accountability and respect (Anderson *et al.* 1997; Respect 2000). Most services have a written programme of work, and programme integrity within the field is generally very high (that is, the groupworkers follow it quite closely). However, delivering effective programmes relies on more than merely following a set course of exercises. The skill of the groupworkers can have a profound influence on the effectiveness of programmes (Andrews 1995; Gondolf 1998; Dobash *et al.* 2000).

This chapter will explore the role of the groupworker in programmes for perpetrators, the ways in which gender affects that role, and the reflexivity and skill needed to maximize the benefit that can be derived from gendering both process and content in the group while simultaneously avoiding the pitfalls. It includes quoted material from interviews with experienced group leaders (2 female, 3 male) and from a group interview with programme attendees to illustrate how the different parties perceive the influence of gender on the groupworker's contribution to the group. It will also draw upon my own background as an experienced practitioner, consultant and trainer in this field of work.

Mixed-gender co-working in perpetrator programmes

Programmes for perpetrators of domestic violence are led, as a rule, by mixed-gender co-working teams. The Respect (2000) guidelines state that this is the preferred model, mentioning two women and one man as a viable alternative. In the early 1990s, there was a good deal of debate between UK practitioners about whether such groups should be run solely by men. Having run groups with other male workers as well as with mixed-gender teams, I have noticed significant differences both for group leaders and for programme participants between all-male groups and mixed-gender co-working.

Groups that are all male tend to express more overt sexism and straightforward misogyny; therefore the belief systems of the men in the programme are more clearly visible. One programme member I interviewed commented: 'If there wasn't a woman on the programme I think we would swear more, use stronger language.' With male workers, there may be greater disclosure of abusive behaviour owing to a lower level of embarrassment or fear of being judged. However, there are a number of disadvantages:

- There is more group bonding around a shared masculinity which is problematic in the context of a groupwork process designed to question gender-based beliefs.
- Groups that are run solely by male leaders fail to give participants the immediate and real experience of engaging in dialogue with a woman about their abusive behaviour and sexism or of learning to do this in a way that remains respectful and acknowledges the damage inflicted by their attitudes to women.
- How the men in the programme respond to the women group leaders is revealing of their attitudes towards women, and this can be used within the group.
- Groupwork that is designed to increase the empathy of men in the programme with the effects of their abusive behaviour on their partners is more emotionally powerful with a woman groupworker.

While programmes run by male workers can be challenging, thoughtful and supportive, the emotional affect is nevertheless reduced by not having a female worker. It is akin to the difference between a group of white people discussing their racism and that same discussion being facilitated by black workers.

> Groups are more serious with (*names female groupworker*). She makes it real and, with the best will and commitment, I can't do that.
>
> (Male groupworker 1)

> Having their behaviour seen by the person who experiences it, they feel judged, there is a projected conscience . . . a sense that it is upsetting for the other person to even hear about their abuse.
>
> (Female groupworker 2)

The roles of the groupworker

There are a number of key aims towards which both group content and process are directed. These are concerned with prioritizing victim safety, challenging denial and minimization, working in an egalitarian and respectful manner, promoting change, teaching critical thinking, developing non-controlling relationships and facilitating empathy. Each is explored in turn below.

Prioritizing safety

The primary focus of the intervention process is to increase the safety of the perpetrators' partners and children. This is one of the areas where there appears to be little difference between the functioning of male and female groupworkers. In practice, prioritizing safety requires the groupworker to

- be aware of the possible negative impact of each aspect of the programme on the group members' partners and children and build in measures to counter these;
- constantly assess the risk that an abuser poses to others and act on that assessment, where necessary, to increase the safety of others;
- participate fully in establishing and maintaining inter-agency protocols that increase the safety of women and children experiencing abuse;
- ensure that the experience of survivors of domestic violence has a continuing role in shaping the way the programme is run and designed.

The programme accepts responsibility towards partners and children as well as group members themselves. With any group that operates not directly with the group it is seeking to empower but with those who are blocking that empowerment (as do many groups in the criminal justice system), there has to be a sense of a contract with the victims and the wider community, beyond the group participants themselves. Women are kept informed, for example, about their partners' membership of and progress through the group, and are specifically told if anything is said which might suggest they are in current danger. They are also given some general background to the programme, including the fact that it is important not to expect too much and not to assume they are safe just because their partners have started to attend a group. As was mentioned above, the Respect (2000) guidelines require parallel support services to be in place for women, and the programme recognizes that some will use this as a safe opportunity to separate. Male and female groupworkers are equally committed to these principles.

Challenging denial, minimization and partner blaming, and maintaining an environment where men can critically explore their abusive behaviour

Challenging denial, minimization and blaming (i.e. projecting blame on to others) forms part of the basic training of any perpetrator programme worker. The initial stage of working with perpetrators is almost entirely about challenging these avoidance mechanisms. It is impossible to maintain an environment where men can critically explore their abusive behaviour within an atmosphere of blaming and minimizing. The groupworker needs to be able to pose questions that bring out the details of a perpetrator's abusive behaviour and the effect this has on his partner, and to keep the focus of the group on ending violence and abuse. How men in programmes react to this often depends on which groupworker is doing the challenging.

Men on domestic violence programmes frequently present their violence as a response to their partners' anger or what they construe as verbal 'attack'. By constructing his actions as defending himself, an abusive man perceives that his partner is to blame for pushing him to react violently. One of the reasons perpetrators find challenges from their partners so intolerable is that they have an exaggerated sense of entitlement (i.e. that their partners just do not have the right to question their authority) (Pence 1999). When a female groupworker challenges them, both she and her male colleague can see this mindset evident in the men's behaviour in the group:

> They don't respond to my comments in the same way, even when I am saying the same thing [as my female co-worker]. Maybe they feel safer, even, when I challenge them. I think they feel more threatened, that it's less justified and more of a slight on their manhood, when it comes from the female worker.
>
> (Male groupworker 1)

> Oh yeah, I can get away with things my female co-worker can't. I can use humour to get something over which the men would hear quite differently from her.
>
> (Male groupworker 2)

> Sometimes I long to be a male worker because everything I say is loaded, or interpreted differently because I am a woman.
>
> (Female groupworker 1)

In order to take a directive and authoritative role in the group, the female group-worker needs to inoculate herself against the anger that can be directed towards her for stepping outside the prescribed female role (Bernardez 1983):

> At times, I don't think the men are able to see that I have a personal insight into their use of violence. They see me as a woman and therefore abused and, therefore, there is some sort of gender war going on and I am just getting at them as men – that I am saying all women are good, all men are bad. It is very easy for them to 'other' me in that way.
>
> (Female groupworker 2)

> I was shocked to see a woman in the group. I thought, 'What does she want? What's she here for?' I thought she must be here because she is a victim of domestic violence herself.
>
> (Man on programme)

An effective female groupworker can use the way the men in the group respond to her as a 'here and now' version of how he behaves towards his partner (Nosko and Wallace 1997). This requires that groupworkers have themselves resolved various issues related to gender, are self-aware and reflective in their own practice, sensitive to their own responses to men in the programme and able to use these to illustrate to participants how they abuse.

Providing a model of egalitarian and respectful ways of relating

Having male and female co-workers in a group offers wonderful opportunities to model an equal relationship and to show that disagreements can be handled non-abusively (see also Chapter 8, this volume). The relationship between the male and female co-workers is constantly on show to the men in the programme. For example, if it looks to the group as if the female worker is the assistant, or if the male worker takes more of the cognitive aspects of the programme, then this will perpetuate the gender myths prevalent in the wider culture about men being in control and more intelligent – which are precisely what the programme is aiming to question.

Co-worker teams develop deliberate strategies to model an equal relationship and alternative forms of male–female interactions to group participants. Often, these are pre-planned attempts to increase the authority of one worker or to present flexible gender roles to the group.

> They seem to sort of take it in turns. One week it's (*names the female worker*) who is grilling you, next week it's (*names the male worker*). They swap around all the time. Sometimes he is playing the woman in a role-play, sometimes she is playing the male. I think they do it so as not to get stereotyped.
>
> (Man on programme)

Often, the male worker will find the men in the group trying to seduce him into being 'matey' with them, isolating his female colleague. Again, he needs to be both aware that this is likely to happen and highly aware of his own gender attitudes in order to resist it. 'They want to share things with me which are not to do with the programme and something they would not do with the female worker' (Male groupworker 1). In perpetrator programmes, it is essential that the male group-worker is the ally of the woman in the room and not of the men. This goes against most of his gender learning and can be an uncomfortable experience for male groupworkers.

> Every so often someone says something about women being nags and will turn to me and say, 'No offence to you.' It feels like a warning that I am the odd one out here. At times like that, I need my male co-worker to come in, or I find myself feeling very isolated.
>
> (Female groupworker 1)

> Working well as a team is a difficult thing to do. I have to keep a distance and resist being part of the male group thing. It's the opposite of what you're supposed to do as a man or what is safe.
>
> (Male groupworker 3)

If the co-workers are not working effectively as a unit then the group's dynamics will be affected, with participants often attempting further to undermine the relationship. The obvious parallels between having a male and a female co-leading the group and many relationship and family structures can be used in understanding the group process, both in debriefing between the workers and in the group sessions themselves.

As well as modelling an equal and respectful relationship with each other, group workers need to respond respectfully to the men in the programme. Listening to men talk about the women they have abused in ways that denigrate and blame them can be a painful experience. Yet all of the challenges to partner blaming and minimization need to be respectful. Groupworkers need to be affirming of the steps the man is taking towards change, while at the same time not colluding with his abuse or minimization of it and remaining mindful of the risk he still poses to others. Being condemnatory of him as a person, as opposed to challenging his conduct, is counterproductive. It triggers defence mechanisms instead of motivating change. Men need to feel supported in working towards a new set of attitudes and behaviours that may be completely unsupported by every newspaper they read, every TV programme they watch and every conversation they have at work or in the pub. The group has to offer them a counterbalance.

Holding out the possibility of change

Following on from the above, groupworkers need the ability to provide for each member of the group a realistic image of the changes each needs to make, even when men in the group do not see that possibility for themselves. Male and female workers say they notice little difference in the general manner in which their co-workers, as men or women, remain supportive of men's change process. All groupworkers, male and female, by using aspects of their own experience and their own critical analysis of that experience, can be helpful to group members. Clearly, though, those experiences do differ by gender, so that precise inputs into the group will vary.

> My male colleagues can use their own experience in ways I can't. I remember this one session on sexual abuse when the group were very resistant to looking at their behaviour in this area and my male colleague talked about some sexually abusive behaviours he had used in his life. Within five minutes, men in the group were beginning to disclose their own abusive behaviours.
>
> (Female groupworker 1)

In the above example, the male groupworker took the risk that none of the other men in the group was prepared to do. He was saying to the other men in the room that using sexually abusive behaviours is common, owing to the social construction of masculine sexuality, and that it is possible to acknowledge this without being hounded out of town as some sort of beast – provided one can see that it was wrong and intends not to repeat it. In this way, and provided he is a critically reflective practitioner, he is able to offer an example of how men can learn to change and deal with difficult feelings positively:

> We were looking at letting go and I used, as an example, the end of my last long-term relationship, which I felt angry and hurt about, but I dealt with that experience – not easily but non-abusively.
>
> (Male groupworker 1)

> If I am using my own experience to illustrate a point in the group, I am very careful that I am doing it because it is useful for the group and not me wanting to be friends with the men.
>
> (Male groupworker 3)

The ability of male workers to use their own experience to aid group process and, by speaking inclusively as a man in the group, to offer an alternative way to live is an option not open in the same way to a female groupworker. Even if she has an equivalent experience she could offer, it would trigger a negative and distancing reaction on the part of the men, such as voyeurism or rejection, rather than a shared journey towards change. Due to the partner-blaming attitudes found in so many of the men on domestic violence programmes, too, any negative conduct the female groupworker may display simply feeds into their prejudices:

> I am very careful what I disclose about my own abusive behaviours. Some of the men in the group get so hooked into seeing women as spiteful and unjust that it's almost like I would be giving them fuel for those beliefs.
>
> (Female groupworker 2)

Frequently, too, the female groupworker is seen as representing all women, which makes her both more and less than just another person in the group:

> There is a kind of authority to what she says. In a really positive sort of way she makes things real and gives the group a woman's perspective on things.
>
> (Man on programme)

It is clearly a strength that the men should start to think about how women perceive situations differently, but it also has dangers. If they are to learn to respect women, they need to see difference and diversity between women and to hear what individual women are saying, not just to assume a homogeneous category of 'woman'. The female groupworker's position can lead to the men in the programme either constructing her as an angry, attacking woman or as the idealized carer (caregiver). Both the idealizing and the demonizing of the woman groupworker is detrimental to the men recognizing the individuality of their partners' experiences and the diversity of women's experience in general and, as such, needs to be made visible to the group.

Enabling men to engage in a critical questioning of their expectations of themselves and the women with whom they have relationships

One of the key ideas underpinning much of the work done with abusive men is that violence is learned behaviour (Bandura 1973; Goldstein *et al.* 1989). Targeting the attitudes and beliefs that support offending behaviours is the cornerstone of all the programmes currently being developed under the 'what works' agenda (McGuire 1995; Taylor-Browne 2001). Programmes for perpetrators of domestic violence engage in similar questioning of attitudes and beliefs but focused on men's understanding, not just of themselves as offenders but also of themselves as men and of their relationships with women. Additionally, perpetrator programmes invite men in the group to engage in questioning the current and past institutional and cultural messages that support their beliefs about gender. For this process work, groupworkers need to be skilled at engaging perpetrators in critical thinking: 'To teach men to think critically a critical process must be created. It must be true dialogue, not simply a pitting of the facilitators against the men in a . . . debate' (Pence and Paymar 1990: 21).

Domestic violence perpetrators have a sense of entitlement in relation to their partners, where the man can set the rules of the relationship (e.g. he can drink, spend money, come and go as he pleases without criticism) and can establish expectations of service (sex, housework, emotional care) from the woman (Blacklock 2001). Even when they admit that their violence is morally wrong, this sense of entitlement allows perpetrators to construct their abusive behaviour as reasonable, given what they see as their partners' unreasonable resistance to their demands. For perpetrators to stop abusing requires them to deconstruct this set of beliefs. The key elements of facilitating this critical thinking for the workers are:

- demystifying notions that gender-based expectations are something innate or natural, as opposed to historical, contextual and changing;
- making visible the intentionality of abusive behaviour;
- posing questions that enable men critically to assess the impact of their gender-based assumptions on their own lives and that of their families;
- remaining inquisitive and interested in discovering how the men in the programme became abusers while retaining the focus of change on the here and now.

Men on programmes who are changing the way they relate to their partners often state that one of the most notable differences is that they are more able to talk to their partners. There is some evidence to support this (Burton *et al.* 1998) and to attest to its importance. Gondolf (1988), in an extensive comparative evaluation of perpetrator programmes, found that one of the most important things men on programmes can develop is the ability to talk things through and to respect their partners' point of view. This was linked with attitude change and, in turn, with their partners noting a greater extent of change and fewer repeat attacks. This suggests that, if a man leaves a programme with the ability to think critically about his own behaviour and to engage with others in that process in an enquiring, open way, then he has acquired some of the tools he will need to build more equal relationships.

> When I can get a group to think through an issue, going from A to B and seeing the penny drop for some, is the most exciting part of the work.
>
> (Female groupworker 1)

For this to occur, the process of the programme needs to be one where group leaders are not trying to win or simply to get the right answers. When groups are didactic, it results in participants who learn to 'talk the talk' but not to 'walk the walk'. This should make programme deliverers wary of over-rigidly following the programme manual that has developed in some offender programmes without doing the work that should underpin or accompany the published exercises.

Male and female groupworkers may differ in how they approach this particular process:

> I am always thinking, 'Where did that [idea] come from? Where did I get that message? How do I benefit or lose through that belief?'
>
> (Male groupworker 3)

> I often think about the impact on the woman as a way to deconstruct an incident. I go to that place more frequently than my male co-workers.
>
> (Female groupworker 2)

The value of having male and female co-leaders working together on perpetrator programmes is clearly demonstrated here, in that each has his/her own relationship to structural gender inequalities. They are able to analyse every situation from different viewpoints, bringing these together creatively in the group.

Enabling the men in the programme to develop new non-controlling ways of relating

Many of the men in perpetrator programmes have been using abusive behaviours for most of their adult lives. The process of change, even for the most motivated of men, is not definitive or linear. A common question asked by men on programmes is, 'Well, if I am not going to be abusive, what else do I do?' Programmes are not about getting men not to feel angry, hurt or resentful – these feelings are part of any relationship – but about enabling men to experience those feelings and yet remain non-abusive. Developing non-controlling ways of relating is not a question of teaching men in the programme the 'right way' to have relationships, but of helping them discover their own strategies, those that will work for them, in respecting the autonomy of their partner and others. Role-play and drama are commonly used in helping men in programmes to develop these non-abusive behaviours.

Male groupworkers have the option of being open about their own struggles in relating respectfully, as discussed above, whereas the female groupworker can offer the men in the programme a chance to develop respectful ways of relating through their relationship with her.

> When we were saying nasty things towards women, she put us straight. . . . I got used to knowing that it's wrong to say that towards women – because I was practising in the group not saying things like that towards a woman it's more reason not to do it at home (Group member's comments in Rex 1998: 13).

Developing the perpetrator's empathy for others, particularly those he has abused

The ability to objectify – to diminish the humanity of – another person seems to be a precursor of inflicting violence on them (Sinclair 1989). A lack of empathy for the impact of their behaviour on their partners and children is a common trait in many domestic violence perpetrators (Dutton 1985; Blacklock 2001). Turning the partner into an object through put-downs and name-calling is one of the reliable predictors of violence towards her (Johnson 1998) and is captured in detail by Hearn (1998) in his study of men talking about their own violence against women. Getting the men on a programme to see their partners as individuals who have their own needs and opinions is one of the key tasks for the groupworkers.

Having a woman worker in the group is important in increasing empathy. When I have run groups with a male co-worker, working on empathy, no matter how well it was done, was not as direct because there was always an emotional distance. At DVIP (the Domestic Violence Intervention Project in London), we often have the woman worker deliver the parts of the programme that give women's experience a voice in the room. The connection with the group is more immediate than when the male worker does this. The downside, as we saw above, is that the woman worker can be seen as representative of all abused women, so we compensate by reversing gender position on other parts of the programme. However, the female worker's role in increasing empathy remains hugely significant.

> They [men in the group] project on to me that I identify with their partners. Therefore it is harder for them to 'other' their partner, as I am somehow her representative in the group.
>
> (Female groupworker 2)

> It is harder to have to talk about your behaviour with a woman, although I feel more comfortable with it now – it adds a touch of reality to it. We are here to work on issues about relating to women and it would be very sterile without her.
>
> (Man on programme)

Conclusion

There has been a clear need to bring in standards of practice for perpetrator programmes and Respect has devoted much of its recent attention in this direction. Yet, over the past few years, I have had concerns that overly prioritizing programme integrity might devalue practitioner skill and that this might result in downgrading also the role of the groupworker. Running programmes is not about mechanically doing what is laid out in a manual. Delivering them well, so that they achieve the most positive outcomes, involves a great deal more than being able to hold firm boundaries, challenge partner-blaming and deliver an educational curriculum. It requires that the group process be vibrant and interactive.

Running an effective programme is about being able to make material fit the participants, not the other way round. Good groupworkers have internalized the programme philosophy – they know the programme content well enough, and are sufficiently comfortable with a range of styles of groupwork to be able to 'go with the moment' if something interesting develops in the group. What they are primarily thinking about in the group is not what comes next in the content (they are steeped in that), but what the men are revealing about their behaviour and attitudes at any particular moment through the process and dynamics of the group. This is the most fruitful material to use to help the men see for themselves, and challenge in each other, what they are saying and doing.

Mixed-gender co-working is a difficult skill to develop. It is acquired by the ongoing analysis of how the male and the female co-worker relate to each other and to the group, in planning and debriefing sessions and through training, supervision and consultancy. The co-working relationship needs time and support to develop. Yet it is a tool that is particularly vital in the delivery of perpetrator programmes because of the gender dynamics these must encompass. One of the obvious major differences between a good programme and a poor one is the quality both of the groupworkers and of their co-working relationship. One good worker cannot compensate for a bad one. Both must be aware, committed, skilled and perfectly in tune with each other, with the group's purpose and with how participants perceive them in the group (separately and together), as well as with their own gender identity. How significant an impact all this has on programme outcomes we do not yet fully know. If, as Gondolf suggests, however, changes in attitude and the use of discussion-based approaches to problems are linked with lowering levels of abusive behaviour, then the ability of the co-worker team to engage men in dynamic explorations of their conduct and attitudes in relationships seems vital to programme success. It is not realistic to expect that exploration to occur unless the groupworkers are engaged in a similar exploration of their own professional relationship as male and female colleagues (Nosko and Wallace 1997). Therefore, valuing the skills and development of co-working teams may well be a key aspect of successful outcomes in programmes for perpetrators of domestic violence.

References

Anderson, G., Colley, D., Hall, R. and Jenkins, A. (1997) *Competency Standards for Intervention Workers: Working with Men who Perpetrate Domestic Abuse and Violence*, Adelaide, Australia: Office for Families and Children, Government of South Australia.

Andrews, D. (1995) 'The psychology of criminal conduct and effective treatment', in McGuire, J. (ed.) *What Works: Reducing Reoffending*, Chichester: John Wiley & Sons.

Bandura, A. (1973) *Aggression: A Social Learning Analysis*, Englewood Cliffs, NJ: Prentice-Hall.

Bernardez, T. (1983) 'Women in authority: psychodynamic and interactional aspects', *Social Work With Groups*, 6, 3/4: 49–63.

Blacklock, N. (2001) 'Domestic violence: working with perpetrators, the community and its institutions', in *Advances in Psychiatric Treatment*, 7: 65–72.

Burton, S., Regan, L. and Kelly, L. (1998) *Supporting Women and Challenging Men*, Bristol: Policy Press.

Dobash, R.E., Dobash R.P., Cavanagh, K. and Lewis, R. (2000) *Changing Violent Men*, London: Sage.

Dutton, L.G. (1985) *The Batterer: A Psychological Profile*, New York: Basic Books.

Goldstein, A.P., Glick, B., Irwin, M.J., Pask-McCartney, C. and Rubama, I. (1989) *Reducing Delinquency: Intervention in the Community*, Oxford: Pergamon Press.

Gondolf, E. (1998) 'Multi-site evaluation of batter intervention systems: how batterer programme participants avoid reassault', Paper presented at the Sixth International Conference on Family Violence, Durham, NH, 12 January 1988, available online at: www.iup.edu/matti/publication

Hearn, J. (1998) *The Violences of Men*, London: Sage.

Iwi, K. and Todd, J. (2000) *Working Towards Safety: A Guide to Domestic Violence Intervention Work*, London: DVIP (PO Box 2838, London, W6 9ZE).

Johnson, H. (1998) 'Rethinking survey research on violence against women', in Dobash, R. and Dobash, R. (eds) *Rethinking Violence Against Women*, Thousand Oaks, CA, London and Delhi: Sage.

McGuire, J. (ed.) (1995) *What Works? Reducing Reoffending: Guidelines from Research and Practice*, Chichester: Wiley.

Morran, D. and Wilson, M. (1997) *Men Who Are Violent to Women: A Groupwork Practice Manual*, Lyme Regis, Dorset: Russell House Publishing.

Mullender, A. (1996) *Rethinking Domestic Violence: The Social Work and Probation Response*, London: Routledge.

Mullender, A. and Burton, S. (2001) 'Dealing with perpetrators', in Taylor Browne, J. (ed.) *What Works in Reducing Domestic Violence? A Comprehensive Guide for Professionals*, London: Whiting & Birch.

Nosko, A. and Wallace, R. (1997) 'Female/male co-leadership in groups', *Social Work With Groups*, 20, 2: 3–16.

Pence, E. (1999) 'Some thoughts on philosophy', in Shepard, M. and Pence, E. (eds) *Coordinating Community Responses to Domestic Violence*, Thousand Oaks, CA: Sage.

Pence, E. and Paymar, M. (1990) *Power and Control: Tactics of Men Who Batter. An Educational Curriculum*, revised edn, Duluth, MN: Minnesota Programme Development Inc. (206 West Fourth Street, Duluth, MN 55806, USA).

Pence, E. and Paymar, M. (1996) *Education Groups for Men Who Batter: The Duluth Model*, 2nd edn, New York: Springer.

Respect (The National Association for Domestic Violence Perpetrator Programmes and Associated Support Services) (2000) 'Statement of Principles and Minimum Standards of Practice', revised version. Master [sic] copy held by DVIP, PO Box 2838, London W6 9ZE.

Rex, S. (1998) *Evaluation Report: Peterborough Pilot Domestic Violence Programme*, Cambridge: Cambridgeshire Probation Service.

Scourfield, J. (1994) 'Changing men: UK agencies working with men who are violent towards their women partners', unpublished MA dissertation, University of Wales, Cardiff, Department of Social and Administrative Studies.

Sinclair, H. (1989) *An 'Accountable/Advocacy' Batterer Intervention Program*, San Rafael, CA: MANALIVE Training Programs.

Taylor-Browne, J. (ed.) (2001) *What Works in Reducing Domestic Violence? A Comprehensive Guide for Professionals*, London: Whiting & Birch.

Chapter 7

Developing the capacity to address social context issues

Group treatment with African American men who batter

Oliver J. Williams

Introduction

The core philosophy about what should be included in batterers' treatment interventions has remained largely the same over the past twenty-five years. These programs tend to incorporate a profeminist historical and social structural critique about male abusive attitudes and behaviors towards women. That is, the abuse of women is an extension of male sexism: the use of power to subordinate, dominate, control, and victimize women. A goal of batterers' treatment and educational programs, to use the US terminology, is to reeducate and restructure abusive men's attitudes and behaviors towards their female partner; and to get them to respond to their female partner in a non-sexist, non-abusive, and non-violent manner.

The field has typically used groups as the mode of treatment, based on a cognitive behavioral approach to counsel and/or reeducate these men (National Research Council 1996). This core profeminist gendered perspective and re-education model remains useful as a framework for reshaping abusive behavior among heterosexual men who batter. But, what this chapter will suggest is important is to expand the content that some men from different backgrounds bring into batterers' treatment and educational groups. Sexism is at the root of domestic violence in heterosexual relationships, but worldviews and backgrounds vary. One model and focus may not be comprehensive enough to address all the concerns and contributors to violence of men who come from different cultures, faiths, countries, customs, traditions and socio-economic statuses, and have different histories. Even though sexism is at the root of violence, how it is manifested among diverse cultures varies. In some instances, the content of the group and the skills of the practitioner are not broad enough to address issues that are seen by some as unrelated to the violence but that are critical in engaging men in developing non-abusive skills (Williams 1999a). The one-size-fits-all model, its application and training, in my view do not incorporate the many manifestations of sexism or other life issues and challenges that result from cultural and social context differences.

It is not my intent to provide an exhaustive critique of batterers' treatment content, models, and perspectives. Rather, this chapter highlights issues that require additional attention and may resonate among certain populations who are less successful in batterers' treatment groups (Bennett and Williams 1999, 2001; Gondolf and Williams 2001). Oppression, poverty, culture, and social context are among the themes that African American men who batter bring to batterers' groups. Familiarity with these themes increases the practitioner's capacity to engage these men by acknowledging the group member's social realities while also confronting problem behaviors. Men in these groups must increase their capacity to address their social context challenges, including those they in turn create for battered women.

Again, the core philosophy and approach for batterers' treatment is as important today as ever before. Choosing to address other content does not presuppose that traditional models are irrelevant; rather, they should be valued and incorporated (Williams 1999b). There is no justification for the abuse of women. Men who batter must not be allowed to use their life experiences to rationalize or justify their violence. But expanding the capacity to address this content seems to me critical in reducing their tendency to displace their anger onto the women they abuse.

Expanding the focus of group treatment

Often African American men in groups discuss long-standing or currently un-resolved issues that seem indirectly related to their violence. Groups can contribute to the re-socialization and education of the client even though not all of the material discussed seems directly associated with partner violence. But the extent to which these secondary issues are addressed depends on how knowledgeable and comfort-able the group worker is in addressing the content men who batter present in-group. For example, a man may want to discuss a challenging issue, perhaps work conflicts with fellow employees or supervisors. Some group workers may feel that this gets men off-track and avoids focusing on the abuse of women. This type of worker would redirect participants to address their relationship with their partners, only. In contrast, other group workers might find such content important. First, they might ask the group member to assess the situation and his behavior with other employees or with his supervisor. Did he handle the situation appropriately? If not, what could he have done differently? Is such conflict a pattern? Group workers and members can help him gain additional insight into the problem and develop appropriate responses, as well as rehearse how to address these types of problem in the future. Second, this group worker could require the man to examine how conflict on the job influences what occurs with his female partner. Was he verbally abusive or physically abusive to her after the conflict at work? Did he blame her for his frustration? When these types of stress occur, is the partner at high risk for physical or emotional abuse? What should be done to handle his problem and not make his partner a scapegoat? How should he inform her about his predisposition? In this case, the group worker facilitates insight through assisting the man in making links between the content at work and his abusive or violent behavior toward his partner. Group workers must develop the capacity to hear the content and help members make connections between their feelings, experiences, and behaviors.

Social context, socio-economic status, and the need for culturally competent services

Some have questioned the effectiveness of group treatment for men who batter but research has indicated that batterers' intervention programs (BIPs) have helped to reduce violent behavior and recidivism (Gondolf 1999a, 1999b). Generally speaking, the men who succeed in such programs tend to mirror the creators of traditional batterers' treatment models: educated, middle-class, and white. Over the last eighteen years, criminal justice intervention, pro-arrest policies, and court-mandated treatment programs have been developed to hold more men accountable for their abuse. Such efforts have increased the numbers of men and particularly poor white men and men of color in BIPs. Men of color tend to be less successful in such programs. African American men do not complete treatment at the same rate as do white males, and their re-arrest rate is also higher (Gondolf and Williams 2001).

Although much has changed over the years, the core philosophy and treatment models have not. The question must be asked, what is missing from conventional approaches that limits the success of poor men and, for the purposes of this discussion, African American men? Cultural competence has been reported as an important consideration in improving outcomes for men of color (Williams 1994a, 1999b; Gondolf and Williams 2001). However, most treatment programs historically have not included cultural competence (Williams and Becker 1994). The following are just a few considerations for practitioners to consider when they conduct batterers' treatment groups that include African American men.

Understanding the influence of oppression, poverty, and social context

Over the last twenty years, the level of violence in the African American community has increased substantially. Some research suggests that family violence is influenced by a person's level of income (Lockhart 1985; Ards 1997). As a group, African Americans are disproportionately poorer than whites. Taylor-Gibbs (1988) notes that, because many of the social supports that had constituted buffers against social oppression for African Americans have been eroded within the last twenty-five years, many community leaders, professionals, and more affluent African Americans have moved to integrated, non-segregated environments. Thus fewer indigenous resources exist within specific African American communities. This has widened the gap in economic diversity, advocacy programs, role models, social supports, social networks and community leadership as well as that between middle-class and poor African Americans (Taylor-Gibbs 1988; Williams 1998). This in turn has created increasingly stressful community living environments, with fewer supports and resources for those who have been left behind (Taylor-Gibbs 1988; Williams 1998). Furthermore, these environments are at increased risk for extreme levels of poverty, frustration, crime, and violence (Taylor-Gibbs 1988; Oliver 1994; Williams 1998). Most African American men and women experience social oppression regardless of social status, but low-income men and women may suffer it more intensely (Gary 1995; Williams 1999b).

Williams (1994b) notes that poor people are not the only group to experience family violence. Clearly, middle-class and upper-class African Americans experience partner abuse as well. Yet the tension associated with social oppression and high-stress community environments may foster conditions that increase the risk for violence in many forms. Codes of conduct and survival may vary from those of people who are unfamiliar with such communities.

It is imperative that practitioners who work with African Americans residing in low-income, high-stress communities should understand their social context and competing challenges. In interviews conducted with community-based human service providers who work in these areas, Williams (in press) reports that many respondents identify such environments as fragile communities. This term characterizes communities, families and individuals whose life experiences and daily living challenges are shaped by their social context and social status in US society. There are a number of factors that shape these challenges: one is racism, but poverty is another. It increases the proportions, concentrations and problems of location of these communities. Poverty contributes to and increases the competing environmental challenges that include, but are not limited to, the following: health concerns such as high rates of infant mortality, low birth weight, teenage pregnancy, poor nutrition, hypertension, diabetes, heart disease, HIV/AIDS, and generally inadequate health care (Cooper-Patrick et al. 1999; Kalichman et al. 1999; Cooper 2001). These communities experience high rates of substance abuse (Well et al. 2001), and higher rates of suicide and interpersonal violence among family, friends, and acquaintances, as well as higher rates of community violence, compared to communities of higher socio-economic status that are also less visible to the law enforcement systems (Hampton et al. 1991, Williams 1999b; Gondolf and Williams 2001).

These communities, which include the poor and the working poor, go hungry and face resource and educational challenges as well as difficulty locating and purchasing adequate housing. They experience high rates of single parenthood, absent fathers or problematic parenting models. They may face unemployment, underemployment, and inadequate transportation, as well as police harassment, profiling or other criminal justice concerns, such as over-representation in public involuntary or correctional systems (Leashore 1981; Wilson 1992; Gary 1995; Li et al. 1999; Saravanabhavan and Walker 1999).

Life in these communities is challenging for women and men. Poverty reduces an abused woman's choices and alternatives. Poor African American women tend to leave and then return to their abusers more frequently, and they tend to need more resources in shelter (Sullivan and Rumptz 1994). They may also stay in violent relationships longer and be more likely to fight back if attacked (Joseph 1995). Homicide at the hands of an African American man is the leading cause of death for African American women aged 15–34. Typically, this is someone very close to her, like a husband or boyfriend. Violent social environments also uniquely affect many African American men. Homicide is the leading cause of death among African American men between the ages of 15–34; they experience high rates of acquaintance violence and suicide.

Some of the men concerned live by a code of the streets that shapes personal interactions under particular conditions (Hawkins 1987; Oliver 1994; Hammond and Yung 1993; Blake and Darling 1994; Roberts 1994; Rich and Stone 1996; Bent-Goodley 2001). These male-to-male attitudes and codes of conduct may extend to interactions with partners, other family members and friends (Williams 1999b). Writers who are concerned about maladaptive behaviors among African American men attempt to discern the social realities and antecedents that produce violence between them without excusing their negative behavior (Nicholson 1995).

When one is exposed to an oppressive structural social context and a hostile living environment, violence and a range of associated maladaptive behaviors are predictable (Staples 1982; Wilson 1992). Although the behavior and the violence are not acceptable, excusable, adaptive, allowable or justifiable, they are predictable. Conventional theories about violence towards women have not included a view through a social context or cultural lens (Williams 1992). Yet both a conventional and a cultural perspective is critical in order to confront the man who batters as well as to create approaches that can more effectively reeducate him, given the challenges, competing issues and rules of his environment. The fact is that, in a trusted group environment, men will discuss the content in their lives. A practitioner must develop the capacity to address such content and relate it back to the man's interactions with the woman he has abused.

The capacity to address content related to a sense of oppression

African American men abuse women for the same reasons that all men do – sexism, and power and control issues (Pence 1989). But, in some instances, I would argue that African American men abuse women as a result of displaced anger due to oppression and social context (Staples 1982; Taylor-Gibbs 1988; Wilson 1992; and Williams 1999b). It is imperative that group workers assist participants to make the connection between oppression and violent behavior. For example, in one treatment group, an African American member explained how he was oppressed in his job. He described how he was a target of ridicule for a group of white co-workers. He explained that the leader of this group was a good friend of his supervisor. In the past, when he had complained, his supervisor had been unresponsive. In the most recent episode, his co-workers had taken the keys out of his pocket and moved his car, without his permission. Then a truck came along and smashed into his car. The man felt that this behavior directed toward him was due to racism. He was very angry and stated he wanted to "go off on somebody."

How should that problem be addressed? Certain workers would feel as though this situation was not relevant to the group. Other workers might feel the situation had merit but deny any racial discrimination or association. A culturally competent worker and group members would know when to acknowledge the racism, when to confront what is not racism, and when to confront violent/abusive behavior. Even if the situation at hand dealt with less extreme and more subtle forms of racism or oppression, the group workers and members would have the capacity to address the issues with the man concerned. In this case, group workers and fellow members acknowledged the racism and helped the man to consider appropriate strategies to negotiate and confront his problem on the job. But a culturally competent group would go much further in examining the dynamics. The group could explore what the man did after the incident. What were his interactions with his partner? Did he displace his anger about the racism onto his partner and, if so, in what ways? If not, how did he manage to avoid doing so? If he did direct his anger at her, what other feelings did he have? Did he feel a sense of powerlessness or frustration? How did he behave toward her? Was he short with her? Did he yell? To what extent did his feelings compare to his states of abusiveness? Was he aware of escalating? Did he hit her? The group members could explore appropriate non-violent and non-abusive ways of interacting with his partner when he feels powerless or frustrated. They could also contribute to improving his and their own insight into teachable moments. That is, the group worker or members could offer the comparison between the group member's feelings of powerlessness, helplessness and frustration due to oppression on the job with how his partner feels when she is the target of his abuse. Practitioners who incorporate this content into the work they undertake acknowledge the man's experiences of racism in society. They explore strategies to assist him to negotiate the conflict. They suggest links between his experiences and his behavior. They also help him make the connection between the oppression he experiences and the oppression for which he is responsible.

High-stress community environments

African American men are uniquely affected by overwhelmed community environments, where they tend to be at high risk for physical harm (Blake and Darling 1994). It is important to recognize that most people in such an environment are operating on a similar set of cognitive and behavioral imperatives. Violence toward women may be one maladaptive behavior that results (Taylor-Gibbs 1988).

Accordingly, when such themes are discussed in BIPs, group workers must be prepared to address the content and make connections with the men's behavior toward their partners. For example, a group member described living in a neighborhood in which he was "fronted off" (embarrassed and challenged) by some male acquaintances. This was a violent environment and these young male acquaintances were trying to force him to join them in harming people in the community. If he did not, they threatened to use violence toward him. He was trying to find a way out of this situation and struggling with the choices: "Do I join with them in violence against others? Do I use violence against them in defense of myself? Do I run away? Can I run away? What about my manhood? Am I really a man if

I don't confront them?" In that situation, the men in the group explained, violence is not the best choice. One member noted the comment of a policeman: "Sometimes people are caught in a circumstance with two bad choices – both can get you into trouble." The group encouraged the man against violence because such a choice could land him in jail. They acknowledged his reality and helped him to examine his options. One message that the man came away with was that it was not unmanly to move away from danger. In this situation, too, the important action, guided by the group worker, was to acknowledge the reality and to confront negative behaviors and choices.

In strictly focused batterers' groups, such content would likely be ignored because it is not directly related to partner violence. Another group worker might acknowledge the situation but merely view it as another example of male social-ization and not an example of social context for some African American men. A culturally competent group worker would acknowledge that this situation is qualitatively different, and that, because a man who batters lacks skill in negotiating these situations, violence could result. He needs help from group workers and members with exploring strategies to assist him to negotiate the conflict in non-violent ways. At the same time, the group would also explore his feelings and actions toward his partner. Did he displace his frustration, fear and anger toward her? When he is faced with difficult situations caused by high stress and stressful choices how does he relate to his partner? Finally, the group would assist the man who batters to make the connection between the oppression he experiences and the oppression he inflicts on his partner.

Understanding the African American batterer brand of sexist themes

African American men should not become overly romantic regarding African Americans' historically egalitarian attitudes toward African American women (hooks 1995; Richie 1996). Both past and present experiences demonstrate that sexism is alive and well in the African American community. Sexism gives all men who batter a license to abuse. This is a common phrase in the field, and it is as true for African American men as for any other racial or cultural group. Many abused African American women choose to remain in an abusive situation because of love, children, family, having nowhere to go, lack of resources, loyalty and/or their understanding of African Americans' experiences with oppression. The woman may see her role as the glue that keeps her family strong and together. Some African American women note that, because of negative stereotypes about the African American family, she is even more committed to keeping the family together (BIHA [Black, Indian, Hispanic, and Asian Women in Action] 1989). Because of their social status experiences and their historical treatment by an unjust criminal justice system, African American men who batter expect that battered women will not cooperate with the criminal justice system when law enforcement intervenes. Regardless of culture, men who batter expect their partners to resist interventions by the criminal justice system. However, the particular experiences of African American men with the criminal justice system, concerning disproportional arrest and incarceration rates, influence African American community perspectives and, generally speaking, make them qualitatively different from those in the white community. Unfortunately, family and community members, too, often expect the woman to subordinate her experiences of her partner's displaced anger resulting from social oppression and a hostile community context, even though she is the immediate target of his frustration due to his sexism (Richie 1996; Williams 1994a). In brief, this describes a specific type of sexism African American women encounter. African American men have experienced oppression, from lynching to racial profiling, but African American women have equally experienced oppression, from rape by slave masters to job discrimination, and are among the truest examples of the feminization of poverty. They also experience sexism from all men, regardless of culture. Negative stereotypes about African American women shape their expectations as to how African American men as well as men and women from other cultures will view, interact and behave towards them (West and Rose 2000). These stereotypes may reinforce internalized racism and abuse by other African American men and women, as well as by men and women from other cultures.

Where domestic violence is concerned, a man's experiences of oppression should not be considered a reason for his partner to tolerate a dangerous relationship. His social context experience may be real, but it does not justify or excuse his abusive behavior towards her. Nor does it explain why she becomes the target of his abuse. Change from abuse to recovery takes time. Women, who remain in such relationships, waiting for change, risk further injury and harm (Williams 1999b). Battered women should be informed about the limits of treatment and that it is not a guarantee of change. If the man does change, it may not be in his relationship with her. Staying is not a guarantee of his ability to change and leaving is not a guarantee of her safety. But, whichever option she chooses, she must maintain a support system and safety plan for use when violence is imminent.

Knowing when to acknowledge and when to dismiss oppression and social context

Just as social learning, male socialization and sexism are explanations for all male violence, social oppression and environmental codes are added explanations for violence among African American men. All men who batter, regardless of culture, are fully responsible for their violent and abusive behavior. It is important to stress that the aforementioned are explanations of, not excuses for, violence. At times, statements concerning racism or the oppression of African American men must be challenged. A culturally competent group worker would know when to confront and when to acknowledge such issues (Williams 1994a; 1994b). Similarly, group workers must prevent collusion among group members on such issues. African American men must be cautioned against attending to racism and oppression to the exclusion of the primary purpose of the group, which is to end violence against women. Group workers must be as aware of men's violence against women as they are of cultural competence.

An imbalance on either issue may result in dire consequences either for battered women or in potential treatment outcomes for men who batter. For example, battered women may be more at risk because group workers have not sufficiently challenged some members to change their behavior; or African American men may disengage from the treatment process due to cultural incompetence on the part of the group worker. In the case examples above, an appropriate way to address the situation would be to acknowledge the racism, then to confront the abusiveness of the man's actions against his partner. Whenever such material is brought to a group, workers can employ this paradigm of inquiry.

Other issues to pursue

This chapter has offered just a few examples of the need for practitioners to expand the content in batterers' groups involving African American men. There are many more issues which could have been included that acknowledge the social realities and challenges of many men who come into treatment. For example, for years we have known about the association between substance abuse and domestic violence (Roy 1982; Bennett and Williams 1999). People in the field of domestic violence have always been clear that substance abuse does not *cause* violence. At the same time, we have been unclear how to address the intersection of these issues. Too often we ignore the drinking or drug use, or we expect the man to get clean and sober before he enters a batterers' group. This inattention assumes that nothing can occur to end his violence unless he is sober first. Is this true? What are the possible alternatives, including addressing both problems simultaneously as tends to happen more in the UK (Humphreys *et al.* 2000.) Is the present way we view the intersection in the USA proof that we are unclear how to proceed?

There are similar undeveloped issues around abusive men as fathers. All battered women want safety and security for themselves and their children. The potential terror from continual torture causes many women to find ways to escape their abusers. Because of the nature of the abuse, common sense would dictate that many battered women and children should sever all contact with the perpetrators. Many women are, indeed, reluctant to reestablish a relationship with their tormentor but are forced by the courts into sharing or giving over custody to the abusive father (McMahon and Pence 1993; Jaffe and Geffner 1998). It is clear that, for many battered women and children, there are not enough safeguards to protect them and the children from the abusive man (Williams *et al.* 2001). Yet, some formerly abusive men *can* be safely involved in parenting. Typically, battered women do want their children to have a relationship with their fathers, provided an adequate standard of safety can be guaranteed from physical and emotional abuse (Mullender *et al.* 2003). There are examples of formerly battered women who are continuing with a dual or co-parenting relationship with the fathers of their children even after the abusive relationship is over. What do we know about women and children who either maintain or reestablish parental connections with men who have abused? What are the conditions under which this can become possible without undue risk? And what are the conditions that strictly prohibit men's association with the women and children they have abused?

At this time there are no clear answers on how to proceed. In the field of domestic violence we must recognize that many men who batter will sustain relationships with their battered partners or children. Because they may continue their abuse or carry the abusive behavior into a new relationship, it seems critical to address the issue of fatherhood in treatment programs for men who batter to reduce their violence towards women and break with social learning patterns to which children may be exposed. Responsible fatherhood organizations have emerged throughout the USA over the last ten years. They work with poor men of color who meet the criteria of "fragile" defined earlier. They address the issues of how to be a nurturing, caring and responsible father. They also address issues concerning unemployment, underemployment, education, and substance abuse. Some are beginning to explore the effect that domestic violence has on children and women. In responsible fatherhood programs and BIPs there is a real opportunity to address the impact of violence on battered women and their children and to teach fathers how to behave with their partners and children in non-abusive ways.

In two examples of domestic violence curricula the goal of the fatherhood sections is for men who batter to identify the ways in which violence can impact on their children, their children's mother, or their partner's children (Williams and Donnelly 1997; Wilson et al. 2000). It is also important for these men to develop appropriate ways to undo the effects of their violence on the children. Men explore how to create non-threatening, non-abusive, non-manipulative, cooperative and respectful relationships with the mothers of their children, regardless of their relationship status (notwithstanding court prohibitions or the women and children refusing contact with him). Again, this is useful additional content that can supplement, but never replace, the mainstream purpose of programmes in confronting abuse and changing men's behavior.

Conclusion

Expanding the content of batterers' groups and the skills practitioners employ within them needs to be further explored. Instead of all batterers being treated with one approach and one focus, perhaps we will begin to develop more specialized models for the intersection of domestic violence and substance abuse or domestic violence and fatherhood. Many battered women's advocates who have been committed to working with poor and abused African American women have expanded their work to include, for example, HIV/AIDS, health care, housing and other issues important to the populations they serve. This is because, as one advocate put it, "These women's lives are very complicated." She felt that if she did not respond to the additional realities of the women she worked with she would not be addressing t he full person. Some of these women are challenged by competing concerns. Domestic violence has a high priority for them, but is not the only issue. This advocate realized that offering integrated supports might be more responsive to women's needs. This may be as true for African American men who batter. To be sure, they need to be confronted and held accountable for their behaviors toward women. But in order for them to change, they may require a different approach or style. We must identify the topics, the style, the content and the approach that will work best in improving outcomes among African American men who batter.

References

Ards, S. (1997) Proceedings from the Institute on Domestic Violence in the African American Community, St Paul, Minnesota: University of Minnesota School of Social Work.

Bennett, L.B. and Williams, O.J. (1999) 'Review of batterers programs' in Hampton, R. (ed.) *Family Violence Prevention and Treatment*, 2nd edn, Thousand Oaks, CA: Sage.

Bennett, L.B. and Williams, O.J. (2001) 'A review of research on batterers treatment', in Renzetti, C., Kennedy-Bergen, R. and Edleson, J., (eds) *Overview of Domestic Violence: Sourcebook on Violence Against Women*, Thousand Oaks, CA: Sage.

Bent-Goodley, T. (2001) 'Eradicating domestic violence in the African American community: a literature review and action agenda', *Trauma, Violence and Abuse*, 2, 4: 316–30.

BIHA (1989) *Broken Promises*, BIHA Minneapolis: Minnesota (video on domestic violence in the African American community).

Blake, W.M. and Darling, C.A. (1994) 'The dilemmas of the African American male', *Journal of Black Studies*, 24, 4: 402–15.

Cooper, R. (2001) 'Social inequality, ethnicity and cardiovascular disease', *International Journal of Epidemiology*, October 30 (supplement 1): S48–S52.

Cooper-Patrick, L., Gallo, J.G., Vu, H., Powe, N., Nelson, C., and Ford, D. (1999) 'Race, gender and partnership in the patient–physician relationship', *Journal of the American Medical Association*, 282, 6: 583–9.

Gary, L.E. (1995) 'African American men's perceptions of racial discrimination: a sociocultural analysis', *Social Work Research*, 19, 4: 207–17.

Gondolf, E. (1999a) 'Characteristics of court-mandated batterers in four cities: diversity and dichotomies', *Violence Against Women Journal*, 5, 1: 1277–93.

Gondolf, E. (1999b) 'A comparison of reassault rates in four batterer programs: do court referral, program length and services matter?' *Journal of Interpersonal Violence*, 14: 41–61.

Gondolf, E. and Williams, O.J. (2001) 'Culturally focused batterer counseling for African American men', *Trauma, Violence and Abuse*, 2, 4: 283–95.

Hammond, R.W. and Yung, B. (1993) 'Psychology's role in the public health response to assaultive violence among young African American Men', *American Psychologist*, 48, 2: 142–54.

Hampton, R., Gelles, R., and Harrop, J. (1991) 'Is violence in black families increasing? A comparison of 1975 and 1985 National Survey rates', in Hampton, R. (ed.) *Black Family Violence*, Lexington, MA: Lexington Books.

Hawkins, D.F. (1987) 'Devalued lives and racial stereotypes: ideological barriers to the prevention of family violence among blacks', in Hampton, R.L. (ed.) *Violence in the Black Family: Correlates and Consequences*, Lexington, MA: Lexington Books.

hooks, b. (1995) *Killing Rage: Ending Racism*, New York: Owl Books.

Humphreys, C., Hester, M., Hague, G., Mullender, A., Abrahams, H., and Lowe, P. (2000) *From Good Intentions to Good Practice: Mapping Services Working with Families Where There Is Domestic Violence*, Bristol: Policy Press.

Jaffe, P.G. and Geffner, R. (1998) 'Child custody disputes and domestic violence: critical issues for mental health, social service and legal professionals', in Holden, G.W., Geffner, R., and Jouriles, E.N. (eds) *Children Exposed to Marital Violence: Theory, Research and Applied Issues*, Washington, DC: American Psychological Association Press.

Joseph, J. (1995) *Black Youth, Delinquency and Juvenile Justice*, Westport, CT: Praeger.

Kalichman, S., Catz, S. and Ramachandran, B. (1999) 'Barriers to HIV/AIDS treatment and adherence among African American adults with disadvantaged education', *Journal of the National Medical Association*, 91, 8: 439–46.

Leashore, B.R. (1981) 'Social services and Black men', in Gary, L. (ed.) *Black Men*, Beverly Hills, CA: Sage.

Li, X., Stanton, B. and Feigelman, S. (1999) 'Exposure to drug trafficking among urban, low-income African American children and adolescents', *Archives of Pediatrics and Adolescent Medicine*, 153, 2: 161–8.

Lockhart, L.L. (1985) 'Methodological issues in comparative racial analysis: the case of wife abuse', *Social Work Research and Abstracts*, 21, 2: 35–41.

National Research Council (1996) *Understanding Violence Against Women*, Washington, DC: National Academy Press.

Nicholson, D. (1995) 'On violence', in Belton, D. (ed.) *Speak My Name: Black Men on Masculinity and the American Dream*, Boston, MA: Beacon Press.

McMahon, M. and Pence, E. (1993) 'Doing more harm than good? Some cautions on visitation centers', in Peled, E., Jaffe, P.G. and Edleson, J.L. (eds) *Ending the Cycle of Violence: Community Responses to Children of Battered Women*, Newbury Park, CA: Sage.

Mullender, A., Hague, G., Iman, U., Kelly, L., Malos, E. and Regan, L. (2003) *Children's Perspectives on Domestic Violence*, London: Sage.

Oliver, W. (1994) *The Violent Social World of African American Men*, New York: Lexington Books.

Pence, E. (1989) 'Batterer programs: shifting from community collusion to community confrontation', in Caesar, P.L. and Hamberger, L.K. (eds) *Treating Men Who Batter: Theory, Practice and Programs*, New York: Springer.

Rich, J.A. and Stone, D.A. (1996) 'The experience of violent injury for young African American men: the meaning of being a sucker', *Journal of General Internal Medicine*, 11, 2: 77–82.

Richie, B. (1996) 'Gender entrapment: when battered women are compelled to crime', in *Proceedings, National Institute on Domestic Violence in the African American Community*, Washington, DC: US Department of Health and Human Services, Administration for Children and Families, Office of Community Services.

Roberts, G.W. (1994) 'Brother to brother: African American modes of relating among men', *Journal of Black Studies*, 24, 4: 379–390.

Roy, M. (ed.) (1982) *The Abusive Partner: An Analysis of Domestic Battering*, New York: Van Nostrand Reinhold.

Saravanabhavan, R. and Walker, S. (1999) 'Prevalence of disabling conditions among African American children and youth', *Journal of the National Medical Association*, 91, 5: 265–72.

Staples, R. (1982) *Black Masculinity: the Black Male's Role in American Society*, San Francisco: Black Scholar Press.

Sullivan, C.M. and Rumptz, M.H. (1994) 'Adjustment and needs of African American women who utilized a domestic violence shelter', *Violence and Victims*, 9, 3: 275–286.

Taylor-Gibbs, J. (1988) *Young, Black, and Male: An Endangered Species*, New York: Auburn House.

Well, K., Klap, R., Koike, A., and Sherbourne, C. (2001) 'Ethnic disparities in unmet need for alcoholism, drug abuse and mental health care', *American Journal of Psychiatry*, 158, 12: 2027–32.

West, C.M. and Rose, S. (2000) 'Dating aggression among low income African American youth: an examination of gender differences and antagonistic beliefs', *Violence Against Women*, 6, 5: 470–94.

Williams, O.J. (1992) 'Ethnically sensitive practice in enhancing the participation of the African American man who batters', *Families in Society: Journal of Contemporary Human Services*, 73, 10: 588–95.

Williams, O.J. (1993) 'Developing an African American perspective to reduce spouse abuse: considerations for community action', *Black Caucus: Journal of the National Association of Black Social Workers*, 1, 2: 1–8.

Williams, O.J. (1994a) 'Group work with African American men who batter: toward more ethnically-sensitive practice', *Journal of Comparative Family Studies*, 25, 1: 91–103.

Williams, O.J. (1994b) 'Treatment for African American men who batter', *CURA Reporter*, 25, 3: 6–10.

Williams, O.J. (1998) 'Healing and confronting the African American man who batters', in Carrillo, R. and Tello, J. (eds) *Healing the Wounded Male Spirit: Men of Color and Domestic Violence*, New York: Springer.

Williams, O.J. (1999a) 'African American men who batter: treatment considerations and community responses', in Staples, J. (ed.) *The Black Family: Essays and Studies*, 6th edn, Boston, MA: Wadsworth.

Williams, O.J. (1999b) 'Working in groups with African American men who batter', in Davis, L.D. (ed.) *A Guide to Working with African American Men*, Thousand Oaks, CA: Sage.

Williams, O.J., (in press) *Poverty and Competing Life Challenges: Working with Fragile Families and Communities around Domestic Violence. Report for the Annie E. Casey foundation*, Baltimore, MD: Annie E. Casey Foundation.

Williams, O.J. and Becker, L.R. (1994) 'Domestic partner abuse treatment programs and cultural competence: the results of a national study', *Violence and Victims*, 8, 3: 287–96.

Williams, O.J., Boggess, J.L., and Carter, J. (2001) 'Fatherhood and domestic violence: exploring the role of men who batter in the lives of their children', in Graham-Bermann, S. and Edleson, J. (eds) *Domestic Violence in the Lives of Children: The Future of Research, Intervention, and Social Policy*, Washington, DC: American Psychological Association.

Williams, O.J. and Donnelly, D. (1997) *Batterers' Education Curriculum for African American Men*, St Paul, MN: University of Minnesota.

Wilson, A.N. (1992) *Understanding Black Adolescent Male Violence: Its Remediation and Prevention*, New York: Afrikan World InfoSystems.

Wilson, S., Donnelly, D., Mederos, F., Nyquist, D., and Williams, O.J. (2000) 'Connecticut's EVOLVE Program', Hartford CT: Court Support Services Division, Judicial Branch, State of Connecticut.

Chapter 8

Gendering work with children and youth

Groups for child witnesses of woman abuse

Susan Loosley and Audrey Mullender

Although direct work with child witnesses of woman abuse is spreading on both sides of the Atlantic (Mullender 1994; Hague *et al.* 2001), and has been positively evaluated (Peled and Edleson 1995; Loosley *et al.* 1997), it is surprisingly easy for it to become diluted and to lose its gendered content. This is because there are competing theories underpinning thinking about violence in intimate relationships. On the one hand, there is a feminist understanding that relates the problem to a fundamental power inequity between men and women in patriarchal society while, on the other, there is a systemic view of relationships as capable of imbalance in either direction within the broader dynamic of the family (see Mullender 1996, Chapter 7, for a fuller discussion). Only where a feminist perspective remains at the fore do a gendered content and process emerge clearly from the group and only in this way are children and young people encouraged to think about what has really gone wrong in the relationships they have witnessed.

As a feminist working in a child protection agency – as a group worker and coordinator of a group work program for children who have experienced woman abuse and for their mothers – one of the authors of this chapter, Susan Loosley, has had the opportunity to address the gendering of these issues with children and youth through the group milieu. Gender inequities and gender stereotyping are common threads throughout the program, funded province-wide by the current Provincial Government in Ontario, Canada. The Community Group Treatment Program for Child Witnesses of Woman Abuse in London, Ontario, is a twelve-week concurrent group program for children and their mothers, where children participate in one group (discussed below) while their mothers (or caregivers) participate in another. Referrals come from all children's and women's services in the city and its rural surroundings, including a shelter (refuge) that specifically serves the aboriginal community. The groups help children from a range of backgrounds to process and understand the violence and abuse they have experienced in the home, while their mothers focus on how best to support the children as they begin to heal from some of the deleterious effects (Jaffe *et al.* 1990; Mullender and Morley 1994). It is our belief and the philosophy of the program that the inclusion of gender issues can contribute towards building healthy egalitarian relationships.

Backing for this view comes from research by the five research centers on violence located across Canada (AFRCV 1999). This overview study identified gaps both in the international and in the Canadian literature, where strategies for prevention and intervention in relation to violence against young women and girls tended to be insufficiently gender specific. In addition, difference and diversity were somewhat neglected, with little content on aboriginal or rural, refugee or immigrant communities, or about young lesbians or disabled girls. Nation-wide focus groups raised issues of devaluing images of women and girls in the media, inadequate responses to sexual abuse and harassment, and, again, an absence of gender-specific anti-violence work. There was a feeling that educational programs needed to span the entire age range and that, unless men's violence was named as the problem, girls could be left to take too much responsibility for learning to keep themselves safe.

This chapter focuses on gendering the content and process of groups with children and youth who have lived with woman abuse. Issues to be touched on include the selection of facilitators and the need for them continually to address and challenge gender issues in co-led groups, the gender content of material utilized in the group, and the gender breakdown of the membership. The main focus, however, will be on examples from Susan Loosley's own experience of including gender content in her work with children and youth in groups for witnesses of woman abuse. This will demonstrate that it is never too early to start alerting children to gender inequalities.

Why is gender an issue when working with children and youth who have witnessed woman abuse?

Children learn their predefined gender roles from an early age and these are reinforced throughout their experience of growing up in their cultural and ethnic group. If the goal of a small group is to work towards healthy relationships, then it is important to look at the gender-role behavior children have already learned in the family. Their gender identity (being a boy or a girl) is deeply embedded in what it means to be male or female in the society in which they live, and they quickly become aware of the different social responsibilities and power resources this opens up (Lipman-Blumen 1984).

In particular, when working with children who have witnessed woman abuse, one immediately comes up against their knowledge of who has power in the family and how to get that power. Again, this takes place within a particular culture and ethnicity (Imam 1994), and is learned at an early age from the abusive role model. It should be noted that this is a more sophisticated statement than the assumption that children who have lived with violence will "grow up like it." While that is a contentious view (see Morley and Mullender 1994 for a summary), it is more readily accepted that both boys and girls may need to learn not to be aggressive and that asserting one's own authority selfishly and jealously over others through all kinds of physical and emotional power play is not an acceptable way of resolving conflict. In promoting healthy relationships, it is important to look at this faulty learning in the wider context of gendered violence, including woman abuse, sexual harassment and dating violence. This, in turn, needs to be considered in the context of a male-dominated society that is oppressive towards women. Yet most prevention and intervention work with children and youth, even in this field, is insufficiently gender specific (AFRCV 1999). It cannot possibly hope to make children re-think what they have observed in the home or in what the media daily presents to them as "appropriate" roles and conduct for men and women.

Throughout history, all the mainstream cultures represented in Canada, the USA and the UK have been promoting a dangerous message: that it is OK for men to dominate and control women. In the media and in the wider society, men are typically portrayed as strong, silent, and powerful while women are stereotypically understood to be passive, sexually available caregivers (Safer 1994a, 1994b). In order for children and youth to begin to address the underlying issues that contribute to violent behavior, they need to explore the gender stereotypes that contribute towards violence against women. Groups for children who witness woman abuse are particularly good forums in which to address gender stereotyping. Both the group work format and the nature of the content enable members to experience the dynamics of relationships and to begin to work together on the issues of gender equality.

How does a feminist perspective inform gender issues when working with children and youth?

We cannot deny the socialization of children and youth (AFRCV 1999) or that socialization is gendered. A feminist perspective gives us the tools to analyse this gender agenda, taking feminism to mean "the comprehensive analysis of the nature and causes of women's oppression" (Jaggar and Rothenburg 1984: xii). Any attempt to dilute gendered issues creates a misrepresentation of the real issue – for example, calling woman abuse "family violence." Groups that operate from a feminist perspective give group members confidence to challenge, in however small a way, the male dominance they encounter outside the context of the group (Butler and Wintram 1991). As a feminist or profeminist group facilitator, one can raise children's and youth's awareness in group of gender inequalities and stereotypes. In so doing, we can potentially work towards healthy egalitarian relationships in a violence-free society.

Gender work with children and youth can begin as simply as in our use of language. Terms such as "policeman" relate to typically male-dominated occupations and suggest that these are exclusionary to women. Thus they contribute to girls' historical experience of not being given equal opportunities. "Police officer," when talking about the professional who may have come to the house in answer to a 911 call, is a more gender-neutral term with which both boys and girls can identify. Children's group workers can continually challenge the language they use in group. This means opting for gender-neutral language in all but one vital regard. The one exception is that we must remain clear that violence in relationships is not perpetrated or experienced equally by men and women. Statistically, and particularly in relation to dangerous patterns of motivation and harm, up to and including homicide, men are predominantly the aggressors (Johnson 1998; Mirrlees-Black 1999). Calling the phenomenon "family violence," "marital violence," or "spousal violence," as if both partners were equally to blame, ignores the power and control that abusive men wield over women. In gender-specific anti-violence work, such as that offered by the program in London, Ontario, the group facilitators challenge themselves and group members in all respects to seek better choices of language and to understand why it is important to do so. As one 12-year-old girl stated in group, "[Using] words that include everyone, including people from other cultures, is the way to be more peaceful" (cited with permission). She captures the larger goal of promoting a violence-free society.

Issues of group content and process

Group facilitators for children and youth understand how women are disadvantaged by power and try to be sensitive to gendered differences in all aspects of group content and process.

Group facilitators

Gender is an essential consideration when selecting group facilitators. For example, some areas of group content may have more impact if facilitated by women, and some group members, for example girls who have been sexually abused by men, may not be ready for a group facilitated by men (Moon *et al.* 2000) as the group members would tend to feel unsafe and mistrusting. Women can better facilitate this work. Conversely, children who have witnessed woman abuse, while also comfortable with women, may benefit from an egalitarian style in a male–female co-led group where the facilitation can model positively for children the sharing of power and control (Pence and Paymar 1990, 1996) inherent in the leadership role. In groups that are co-led by a male and a female facilitator, provided that co-workers are thoroughly prepared and can work effectively together, there is the potential continually to address and challenge gender issues. This can help children better to understand the lower status imposed on women by abusive partners and in the wider society: "The lower social status of women relative to men is a major cultural factor in why men abuse women" (Grusznski *et al.* 1988: 440). Facilitators may inadvertently reinforce stereotypical sex roles by assuming that these are the basis for healthy functioning. Yet the family is one of the places where women are most oppressed and children are socialized into inequality (Lipman-Blumen 1984). Feminist group workers continually examine gendering in the context of other culturally based assumptions and processes (De Chant 1996). They provide children and youth with a feminist value system that addresses the harmful effects of gender stereotypes.

In a female–male co-led group, children can benefit from identifying with the group worker of the same sex as themselves, while clarifying problems, issues or concerns with the worker of the opposite sex. The activities and group format should be designed in such a way that female and male group leaders equally share in challenging gender stereotypes and gender inequities, so as to "convey a positive message about women and egalitarian relationships" (Grusznski *et al*. 1988: 440). At the same time, activities that focus on gender roles will enable children to examine their own roles within their families and with their peers. Broadening children's own perspective of themselves may improve their self-esteem, which is an essential goal of the group.

In the London, Ontario, groups for children who have witnessed woman abuse, the program organizers have valued co-leadership by peaceful, nurturing, caring, progressive men. In groups where men participate, equal sharing of power and positive conflict resolution are modeled for the children. It is interesting, for example, when the leaders engage in a mock conflict of ideas in front of the children, the group members look on wide-eyed. The workers wondered initially whether the children expected violence to occur. After reviewing the conflict and its resolution with the members, the children clarified that they did not in fact expect violence but, rather, were looking for the warning signs to indicate that there was a power imbalance between the co-leaders and whether the person with power was going to be abusive (for example, verbally abusive and dismissive). This was discovered by a brainstorming exercise on what the warning signs could have been to indicate that violence or abuse of power might occur. Observing, instead, mutual respect and a calmly negotiated resolution was an important lesson for the children, showing that it is possible to disagree without becoming oppressive.

Despite the potential benefits of mixed-gender co-led groups, currently most group workers are women. Only one group out of twenty a year is co-facilitated by a woman and a man. In a similar program for families who have experienced woman abuse – the Anti-Violence Program at the Family Service Center of Ottawa, Carleton – only women facilitate the groups, though that is a matter of practice rather than of principle. Both programs would be happy to accept as co-workers profeminist men who are knowledgeable of issues of woman abuse and the effects on children. In contrast, neither program would support men as group workers for the mother's group, where all the members have been recently abused by men.

Group material

Gender is an issue when selecting group material because "conducting such work in a gender-neutral context creates an illusionary level playing field for all participants" (AFRCV 1999: 12). Unless it is made clear to young people that violence in the home is embedded in gender inequality, they will take away misleading messages about what human beings need to do to live free of violence in their intimate relationships. Girls will assume too much of the responsibility (expecting to have to conform to male demands when they grow up), while teenage boys' greater tendency to tolerate the abuse of women in society (Mullender *et al.* 2003) will be challenged too little. If we are to take the different socialization of girls and of boys into account in planning this work, the material needs to be gendered.

The manual *Group Treatment for Children Who Witness Woman Abuse: A Manual for Practitioners* (Loosley *et al.* 1997) is clearly gendered, identifying violence in the home as primarily the abuse of women by men. Activities such as watching a movie that features woman abuse by a man, from the children's perspective, addressing myths about men's violence, and considering how men need to take responsibility for their abusive behavior are among the gender-specific examples used in group. An example of how easy it is to slip out of this gender awareness, however, is provided by the manual for pre-school children *No Violence = Good Health* (Foote 1998), which was closely modelled on Loosley *et al.*, yet waters down the content and refers to woman abuse as "family violence."

Composition of the group

In order to create an appropriate context for gendered material, group membership is usually mixed, with approximately half the group being male and half female. A constant flow of referrals makes it possible to maintain this balance, even though the groups are divided relatively narrowly by age, with an age span of only two or three years in each. A workable alternative is to have same-sex membership, and this has occasionally happened but is not the norm. It is not acceptable to have a group with only one girl or one boy and, say, seven members of the opposite sex. This is particularly important for girls, since isolation in the group could compound that already experienced in society and might mean that the group experience would not be beneficial. It does appear that, in younger groups, from the age of 4 or 5 up to about 9, the sex of members appears to be less of an issue. Above this, up to the program maximum of 16 years, members themselves highlight gender issues in group composition from the very beginning, for example by opting to sit with others of the same sex.

Examples from the groups

The examples that follow show how gender-specific content straddles all the age groups served by the program.

Gender-neutral language

It is never too soon to begin addressing gender issues. In groups for pre-school children, in the age band 4–6 years, members already have well-established assumptions about what is appropriate for men and women and they already unthinkingly use gender-specific language. This can provide an excellent opportunity to challenge gender attitudes, both as these are expressed in the group and as they reflect the wider society and the rightful place of men and women within it. When asked what their parents do, for example, a child – we'll call him Sean – might respond, "My dad's a garbage man." The facilitators, who need to have undertaken careful pre-planning in order to be ready to work together when this opportunity arises, open this up into a story. "I knew a mummy once who collected garbage and worked on a garbage truck, like your daddy. What would we call her?" The children, turning "garbage man" into its gendered alternative, might reply with such suggestions as "garbage lady" or "garbage woman." One of the workers then asks, "Can we think of a word that doesn't have to be a mummy or a daddy, but just anyone who does that job? If they collect the garbage, for example, could we call them a 'garbage collector'? Then this woman I know is a garbage collector and Sean's daddy is a garbage collector too." If this exchange were taking place with 6–8 year-olds, who have more experience of life and a greater tendency to talk back to the facilitators, one of them might well protest at this point, "But I've only ever seen a man doing that job." Again, this provides wonderful material to take the discussion further, for example by asking, "Does that mean a woman can't do the job? Why not?" If the children think that the work is too heavy and a woman not strong enough, one of the facilitators will say, "Let's think of all the things your mummy lifts," eliciting a list such as "the shopping," "the baby's stroller," "me!" This establishes that women are actually quite strong. The same steps can be used to prove that they also do plenty of dirty jobs. It is important, with these younger children, to keep the ideas simple and to the point. It is also crucial to return as often and as naturally as possible to the topic of woman abuse. For example, abusive relationships are typically based on expectations of hyper-rigid gender roles and a connection could be made to these, particularly if the group has already discussed them.

The facilitators also model non-stereotypical, non-gender-specific, and non-hierarchical roles wherever possible. For example, care may be taken to have the man putting out the snack for the children and to ensure that the female facilitator takes a lead on at least half the exercises.

Challenging power

With elementary school-aged children, between the ages of 7 and 11 (which would normally span more than one group), it can be particularly important to teach them how to challenge power safely, including in their assumptions about themselves. The facilitators, again with pre-planning so that both are watching out for an opportunity, may set up a role-play or a scenario in a way that the girls get to be leaders and can teach the boys in the group. For example, in a safety planning activity in the group, where dolls in a dolls' house are being used to represent parents arguing and Dad is starting to hit Mum in the kitchen, the children are asked to suggest where in the house would be a safe place to go while the violence is happening. This could be in their own room, under the bed, or wherever they would be safest. The children are encouraged to identify closely with the exercise so that they apply the learning to themselves, for example by having dolls available to represent a range of ages and ethnicities and asking children to model the constellation of their own family with the dolls they select.

Once the enacting of the violent attack has started, the group workers encourage the children to focus on the feelings they had when this kind of thing went on in their own homes. The doll-child may be imagined as frightened and crying. A facilitator will ask, "How can we comfort this young kid who's crying?" A boy might try to hug the doll and put her back in her bed. As most girls have more skills in holding and nurturing a doll-baby, so the group worker asks, "Sally, can you show me how *you'd* put her back in bed," so that Sally is now teaching the boys in the group how to do the task gently and with sensitivity. Provided it is something the worker knows Sally will be good at, or has observed her doing well in the group (painting, drawing, or whatever), it need not be a stereotypically female activity that Sally teaches. In any case, she is modeling it for boys, who are asked to copy what she does and to try and do it as well as she does, so the exercise is cutting across two gender stereotypes in teaching boys to be nurturing and in putting Sally in the limelight as a person with abilities and strengths that are worthy of emulation.

Another example would be drawing the power and control wheel (Pence and Paymar 1990) and asking a question such as, "How do we know using male privilege (or intimidation or emotional abuse) is abusive behavior?" If a boy is not sure, the worker can get a girl to tell him. In this subtle way, both sexes learn that girls have resources and knowledge that give them the power to promote gender equality in the group.

Co-operative games

With children of around 9–11, cooperative games can be a useful way of challenging gender role assumptions. This need not even take place in the formally convened group as such. For example, a facilitator arriving one week saw that a small group of children – two boys aged 9 and 10 and a girl of 10 – had got out the Monopoly board and were going to play until the others arrived for the start of group. The worker immediately and nonchalantly suggested that the girl be the banker, in such a subtle fashion that this adult intervention in a game they had initiated themselves went unremarked by the children. Mika, as we will call her, protested, "Oh, I've never been the banker before," to which the facilitator responded, "I know you can do it. Let me just show you how to get started," and spent a couple of minutes teaching Mika what she needed to do. Thus Mika found herself controlling the group's money, something neither she nor either of the others had ever seen their fathers allowing their mothers to do. The game only lasted for fifteen minutes and took place in the "dead time" before group started, yet it contained within it an important message. That Mika made a very good banker, getting all the amounts right, also boosted her self-confidence and increased her credibility with the group.

Once again, this example clearly demonstrates how essential it is that the group facilitators are ready to seize any opportunity to make a gendered point to the children. Much of the planning and debriefing, before and after group sessions, concentrates on the group workers' and group members' gender roles so that no chance is missed to portray girls as skilful, as leaders, as teachers, and as able to occupy positions of power. Similarly, language is scrutinized to ensure that it conveys messages that will challenge what children have learnt to regard as an unchanging reality about gender roles and male–female behavior.

Ripples from the group: identifying and problem-solving around anger

Evidence that lessons from the group are applied to children's lives outside it came from an 11-year-old girl we will call Maria. Maria copied something from the board at school and brought it to group to be raised in discussion. A male teacher had written up the words "Girls are pretty and wear nice clothes. Boys are smart and strong." His original pedagogic purpose is lost to us now, but may well have had something to do with the use of language and nothing to do with content. Nevertheless, Maria, remembering what she had been learning in the group for child witnesses of woman abuse, was unhappy at being asked to copy out these statements in class and brought the matter to group to ask the other children and the facilitators what she should do. The group helped her to figure out that she would not feel comfortable talking to the male teacher about what had happened, but that she could raise it with her mother. Her mother rang the group facilitator and problem solved the issue by talking about it and working out what to do. She then went to Maria's teacher and to the principal of her school to challenge what had been presented as acceptable learning material for Maria and her classmates, and was successful in eliciting a letter of apology.

The facilitators were delighted that Maria had thought of bringing this material to group and that she had felt able to do so. They were also pleased that the group had dealt so well with the question Maria had posed. In the wider discussion that the example provoked, the children worked out that intelligence and strength, on the one hand, and good looks and nice clothes on the other, are not even opposites. They attribute positive qualities to boys but an attractive outer appearance only to girls. This opened up a useful discussion about how damaging stereotypes can be and how important it is to challenge them, as well as ways in which this can be done. Maria had been particularly upset and offended that she was expected to write down the words she objected to, as part of a lesson at school. Once again, we see the facilitators primed to seize an opportunity that presented itself, out of the blue, to reinforce and extend learning about sex-role stereotypes. Had they been rigidly following the manual, they might have brushed this aside as preventing them from covering that week's planned material. Instead, they saw it as a great opportunity to use something real, from the children's own experience, to engage with the latter's feelings of anger and powerlessness and to help them realize that there are ways to take control and to move forward, even with an authority figure like a teacher.

The wider lessons for the children were that the group was a safe place to disclose gendered information that made someone feel uncomfortable, that they could use the group to identify and tackle stereotyping, that the group could help its members to problem solve, and that it is important to identify how something makes you feel before you do anything about it. In this case, Maria felt resentful and angry but, once she recognized this, with the help of the group she was able to do something about it. The earlier work undertaken in group on gender stereotyping and on recognizing and dealing constructively with anger had taken root with Maria, and the children had all been able to use their learning positively. The group program manual, for example, has an "anger exercise sheet" with the following statements to complete:

1   When I am angry I usually feel ——
2   When someone gets angry with me I usually ——
3   I get angry when ——
4   List three things that you can do to help you calm down when you are angry
     ——

(Loosley *et al.* 1997: 64)

It also has a problem-solving exercise broken down into the following stages:

Step 1:   What is the problem?
Step 2:   What are some solutions?
Step 3:   For each solution ask:
            Is it safe?
            How might people feel?
            Is it fair?
            Will it work?
Step 4:   Choose a solution and use it.
Step 5:   It is working? If not, what can I do now?

(Loosley *et al.* 1997: 65)

These were the steps the group used to help Maria solve her problem at school, and they are equally useful for living violence-free in interpersonal relationships.

Act like a man/be ladylike

The program uses a particularly good activity from the manual *Healthy Relationships: A Violence Prevention Curriculum* (Safer 1994a, 1994b) called "Act Like a Man/Be Ladylike Stereotypes" with children in their early teens. Initially, the group learns together that a stereotype is "an assumption that a person will have certain abilities, characteristics, behaviors and values just because they belong to a certain race, gender, religion, social class, family etc." (Safer 1994a: 12). The group leaders next write "Act like a man" on one sheet of flipchart paper and "Be ladylike" on another, before displaying both on the wall. Group members are asked to generate a list of what it means to act like a man. The list often includes terms such as: "tough," "in control," "don't cry," "leader," "strong muscles," "sports player," and so on. After drawing a box around the list, the facilitators identify it as being the male stereotype. They then do the same for the "be ladylike" page which often generates terms such as "nurturer," "thin," "pretty," "virginal," "passive," "care giver" and "quiet." After drawing a box around this second list, the facilitators identify it as being the female stereotype. They then use both lists to look at what perpetuates stereotypes and what happens if someone does not fit into what is in the box. The children in group are readily able to volunteer the slang names thrown at people who do not fit in. For example, a boy or man may be identified as "weak," "wimp," "nerd," "gay," "loser," "a woman," "useless," and so on. Girls or women may be called "bimbos," "sluts," "butch," "tomboy," "a bad mother", and many other names. A tremendously lively dialog occurs around this activity, and it can readily be linked to woman abuse through the rigid role expectations abusive men tend to have of themselves and their partners, together with the myth that violent men are "real men" who can show affection only through jealousy and brutality. When looking at what reinforces these gender stereotypes, group members have identified parents, the media, movie and fictional characters such as Rambo or Cinderella, sports, soap operas and magazines. The activity provides an unfailing opportunity for group members to challenge and address gender stereotypes within a family, their community and the wider social context.

Challenging myths

With teenagers, in groups for those aged 12 and above (again, spanning more than one group within this age range), the "Myths" game is popular (Loosley *et al.* 1997). The game is based on a series of flashcards bearing statements with which participants are invited to agree or disagree, such as "Pregnant women do not get abused by their partners," or "If a woman did not like the abuse, she could easily leave." Although it is played in teams, "Myths" is not a competitive game and no points are awarded. The purpose of it resides in the discussion to which it gives rise. One of the cards, bearing a common myth about woman abuse, is offered to a member of the team to read out and say something in response to questions such as "Why is that a myth?" The game can lead to discussion around ideas presented in the media, for example in the lives of well-known figures who have experienced abuse, such as Pamela Anderson, or who have been personally abusive, such as Mike Tyson.

Teens are ready to think through the questions in more detail, and it is important to raise issues with them about their own dating relationships since this is the other sphere in which they will be seeing inequality and quite possibly abuse, if not personally then among their friends (Price *et al.* 2000). As girls become readier to show their aggression in society and to retaliate if abused, a boy may say in group, "I've been hit by a girl," though discussion might reveal that the relationship was already abusive in other ways and that his girlfriend was fighting back rather than initiating conflict. Thus the boy is minimizing his partner's experience of his own behavior and attitudes. Girls, on the other hand, even when they act big and tough, may come to realize that they are still not the ones with the power in the relationship. Other areas that frequently come up include fashion, sexuality and partner choice. Girls say they dress skimpily because they want to. Boys say they like looking at girls dressed like that. The facilitator may ask the girls, "What do you want boys to like you for?", and the boys "What kind of girlfriend do you want?" This reveals that the basis of a sound and lasting relationship has little to do with looks, even though boys may find it hard to get past saying – even if they want to go out with a smart girl, someone who's intelligent – that "She's gotta look good." Homophobic and heterosexist assumptions can be challenged through discussion of youth who choose partners of the same sex.

This discussion can also lead into reinforcing work in the group on who is responsible for violence. If a girl dresses provocatively, or "leads a boy on," he may argue that she is partly to blame if she is sexually assaulted or hit when she says "No!" It is a crucial aim of the group, with all age groups, to teach children and youth that the perpetrator must take responsibility for his own violence. This lesson has certainly not yet been learnt by the wider population of young people. In the UK, for example, one-third of teenage boys in a recent research study agreed with the statement "Some women deserve to be hit" (Mullender *et al.* forthcoming). The London, Ontario, group program as a whole undertakes a considerable amount of work on helping members to be clear that their mothers were not to blame for being abused and that they, the children, had no part in it, either, even if the abuser implicated them in some way such as making them watch, threatening to harm them in order to force compliance from their mother, or using them as an excuse for picking an argument with her. Over time, most children who live with woman abuse do come to recognize that the perpetrator was to blame and that he must take responsibility for his own actions (Mullender *et al.* forthcoming).Violence prevention work can take these issues wider and can be linked with general anti-violence efforts in school as well as in group, including those around bullying and racial abuse and harassment, without losing its gendered content.

Conclusion

It is vital that group leaders for children and youth critically challenge themselves to dialogue honestly and meaningfully about gender, despite their anxieties about the potential backlash related to this topic. Indeed, being comfortable with acknowledging and affirming gender differences will help all of us to realize how much our strengths lie in our diversity. Such a commitment will foster personal and professional growth among group workers for children and youth and enable them to take a step in the direction of ending violence against women. Children who have grown up with violence and abuse observe, at home, a modeling of an unacceptable polarity in gender roles. Group work programs such as the one discussed here can help them to challenge this faulty learning and to grow up healthier and happier. Consequently, there is a need for training and research to focus upon this area so that future practice can be well supported.

References

AFRCV (Alliance of Five Research Centers on Violence) (1999) *Violence Prevention and the Girl Child*, London, Ontario: AFRCV.

Butler, S. and Wintram, C. (1991) *Feminist Groupwork*, London and Newbury Park, CA: Sage.

DeChant, B. (1996) *Women and Group Psychotherapy: Theory and Practice*, New York, NY: Guilford Press.

Foote, K. (ed.) (1998) *No Violence = Good Health: A Group Program Manual to be Used with Pre-School Aged Children Who Have Witnessed Family Violence*, London, Ontario: Merrymount Children's Center.

Grusznski, R.J., Brink, J.C. and Edleson. J.L. (1988) "Support and education groups for children of battered women," *Child Welfare*, 67, 5: 431–44.

Hague, G., Kelly, L. and Mullender, A. (2001) *Challenging Violence Against Women: The Canadian Experience*, Bristol: Policy Press.

Imam, U.F. (1994) "Asian children and domestic violence," in A. Mullender and R. Morley (eds), *Children Living with Domestic Violence: Putting Men's Abuse of Women on the Child Care Agenda*, London: Whiting & Birch.

Jaffe, P.G., Wolfe, D.A., and Wilson, S.K. (1990) *Children of Battered Women*, Newbury Park, CA: Sage.

Jaggar, A.M. and Rothenberg, P.S. (1984) *Feminist Frameworks: Alternative Theoretical Accounts of the Relationships Between Women and Men*, 2nd edn, New York: McGraw-Hill.

Johnson, H. (1998) "Rethinking survey research on violence against women," in Dobash, R.E. and Dobash, R.P. (eds) *Rethinking Violence Against Women*, Thousand Oaks, CA, London and New Delhi: Sage.

Lipman-Blumen, J. (1984) *Gender Roles and Power*, Englewood Cliffs, NJ: Prentice-Hall.

Loosley, S., Bentley, L., Lehman, P., Marshall, L., Rabenstein, S., and Sudderman, M., (1997) *Group Treatment for Children Who Witness Woman Abuse: A Manual for Practitioners*, London, Ontario: Community Group Treatment Program (available from: Children's Aid Society of London and Middlesex, P.O. Box 7010, London, Ontario, Canada N5Y 5R8).

Mirrlees-Black, C. (1999) *Domestic Violence: Findings from a New British Crime Survey Self-Complete Questionnaire*, Home Office Research Study No. 191, London: Home Office.

Moon, L., Wagner, W. and Kazelskis, R. (2000) "Counselling sexually abused girls: the impact of the sex of the counsellor," *Child Abuse and Neglect*, 24, 6: 753–65.

Morley, R. and Mullender, A. (1994) "Domestic violence and children: what do we know from research?" in Mullender, A. and Morley, R. (eds), *Children Living with Domestic*

Violence: Putting Men's Abuse of Women on the Child Care Agenda, London: Whiting & Birch.

Mullender, A. (1994) "Groups for child witnesses of woman abuse: learning from North America," in Mullender, A. and Morley, R. (eds) *Children Living with Domestic Violence: Putting Men's Abuse of Women on the Child Care Agenda*, London: Whiting & Birch.

Mullender, A. (1996) *Rethinking Domestic Violence: The Social Work and Probation Response*, London: Routledge.

Mullender, A., Hague, G., Imam, U., Kelly, L., Malos, E., and Regan, L. (2003) *Children's Perspectives on Domestic Violence*, London: Sage.

Mullender, A. and Morley, R. (eds) (1994) *Children Living with Domestic Violence: Putting Men's Abuse of Women on the Child Care Agenda*, London: Whiting & Birch.

Peled, E. and Edleson, J.L. (1995) "Process and outcome in small groups for children of battered women," in Peled, E., Jaffe, P.G. and Edleson, J.L. (eds) (1995) *Ending the Cycle of Violence: Community Responses to Children of Battered Women*, Thousand Oaks, CA: Sage.

Pence, E. and Paymar, M. (1990) *Power and Control: Tactics of Men Who Batter. An Educational Curriculum*, rev. edn, Duluth, MN: Minnesota Program Development Inc. (206 West Fourth Street, Duluth, MN 55806, USA).

Pence, E. and Paymar, M. (1996) *Education Groups for Men Who Batter: The Duluth Model*, 2nd edn, New York: Springer.

Price, E.L., Byers, E.S., Sears, H.A., Whelan, J., and Saint-Pierre, M. (2000) *Dating Violence Among New Brunswick Adolescents: A Summary of Two Studies*, Research Paper Series No. 2, Fredericton, New Brunswick: University of New Brunswick, Department of Psychology and Muriel Fergusson Centre for Family Violence Research.

Safer, A. (1994a) *Healthy Relationships: A Violence Prevention Curriculum. Grade 8: Gender Equity and Media Awareness*, 2nd edn, Halifax, Nova Scotia: Men For Change.

Safer, A. (1994b) *Healthy Relationships: A Violence Prevention Curriculum. Grade 9: Forming Healthy Relationships*, 2nd edn, Halifax, Nova Scotia: Men For Change.

Chapter 9

Genderbending

Reflections on group work with queer[1] youth

Kate DeLois

As usual I was running late and parking places were scarce. It was damp, drizzly, and already dark at a few minutes before seven on this early fall evening in New England. Giving up on a parking space anywhere near my destination, I parked in a slightly illegal spot, locked the car and hurried the few blocks to the building. As I turned the final corner I was confronted with a menacing-looking group of teenagers. Dressed in black leather jackets, torn jeans, hair sprayed all the colors of the rainbow, piercings sprouting from eyebrows and lips, their features were difficult to make out in the coagulating fog from the bay and the cloud of cigarette smoke that engulfed them.

I drew closer and was greeted warmly.

"Hey, Kate, got the keys?"

"Yep, right here," I replied, displaying a keychain. "Coming up?"

"Sure, we'll be there as soon as we finish these butts."

"OK," I said, and continued towards the building. As I unlocked the door I was greeted by another, smaller, knot of teens.

"Hey, glad you're here. We were starting to get cold," one undersized girl in a lightweight denim jacket said. Her lips were blue, giving credence to her claim of hypothermia. Oh, I realized. That was lipstick, matching her fingernails.

The smaller group of four joined me in the elevator ride to the top floor. I unlocked the final door, turned on the lights and then we set about arranging the room for our Friday night support group. Chairs were placed in a circle and snacks appeared from the cupboard.

"Who's on with you tonight?" queried one young man.

"Pete," I replied. "But he said he'd be a bit late, so we'll get started without him."

Another fellow, who I recognized as Chuck, said, "Cool. I like Pete." He stuffed some condoms in his pocket, taken from one of the baskets placed strategically around the room, and headed for the cookies.

As we waited for the rest of the group to join us I looked around the room. A poster on the wall proclaimed "Gay Pride." Another showed two men embracing, while warning "Safer Sex Means Never Having to Say You're

Sorry." Pink triangles and rainbows were a major part of the decorating theme. Sign-up sheets for committees, political activities, and social events dotted the walls. This was a safe space for gay, lesbian, bi, trans and questioning (g/l/b/t/q) youth. For some, the support group afforded the only two hours in the week when they were in a place where they felt that safety. Every time I came here I was filled with gratitude that this program existed – and also with sadness that it had to.

The smokers joined us and after some initial joking, bantering and greetings we settled into our chairs to begin. The opening ritual consisted of reading the mission of the organization, "to create a safe and supportive environment for gay, lesbian, bi, trans and questioning youth," followed by a reading of the ground rules. A large laminated copy of the ground rules was passed from hand to hand and each person read one of the rules aloud. "No side conversations" . . . "What is said in the meeting stays in the meeting" . . . "No shame, blame or guilt."

At the conclusion of the ground rules, check-in began. An eager young man named Phil jumped in.

"I'll go," he said. "My name is Phil, and this past week was hell. I had a fight at school, my mother has been ragging on my ass for days, and Jason and I broke up."

He went on to detail the events of the week at great length until Jasmine broke in, "Hey, Phil, it's been rough and we're sorry and all, but how about leaving some time for the rest of us?"

"Uh, sure, sorry," a red-faced Phil responded.

The guy next to him reached over and patted his shoulder as Jasmine began her check-in.

This was a typical Friday evening at YouthPride, an organization devoted to providing g/l/b/t/q youth with a safe space to gather, share experiences, and interact with adult volunteers who serve as role models for this otherwise marginalized segment of the youth population. In the time I had been associated with the organization it had grown from a once-weekly support group, staffed entirely by volunteers, that met in a space shared with another social service organization, to a dynamic agency, staffed by professional social service workers, offering outreach, support, education and social and political activities every night of the week. Located in the heart of the downtown of a small New England city, YouthPride drew youth from all over the southern portion of the state and was the model for similar organizations that had begun to sprout up in other parts of the state.

There is a general belief that the g/l/b/t population is a "community." The "gay community" or the "gay agenda" are talked about both within the queer population and among our political allies and foes. The idea of a "gay agenda" has always made me chuckle. Anyone who knows us knows that we can't agree on *anything*, let alone a whole agenda. We are no more monolithic than any other segment of the population, but often our diversity and differences are overlooked for the sake of political unity or simplicity. Consider, for example, high-flaming drag queens and radical feminist lesbian separatists and you begin to see the difficulty. To the heterosexual world, these two extremes might belong to one category called "queer." To the rest of us, frankly, it's sometimes hard to make the connection. One of the major differences, and one that is difficult to discuss, is *gender*. It is difficult to discuss because to a large extent queerness is about challenging gender as it is constructed in our culture. Queerness is about gender-bending, and even about challenging our understanding of sex as a biological category. One of the great freedoms that comes with being queer is the permission we give ourselves to appear and behave in "gender-inappropriate" ways, in other words to give expression to a full range of human behavior, attitudes, emotions, and outward appearances rather than constricting ourselves within rigid gender roles.

More than in "straight" society, the queer community encompasses the full continuum of very "masculine" men and women, androgynous men and women, and very "feminine" men and women. Those with "gender-appropriate" mannerisms and appearances are the least visible to society at large and in turn are the least threatening to societal gender norms. On the other hand, "feminine" men and "masculine" women seem to jar society's sensibilities to the point where these individuals are at high risk for verbal and/or physical assault. Visibly queer folks serve the function of helping society define the boundaries of what it means to be male or female. The social sanctions which arise in response to crossing those boundaries in the US include the denial of: federal civil rights, open service in the military, and the legal right to marry with its attendant privileges (such as being designated as the legal next of kin in the event of serious illness or death, immigration, etc.). In addition to these institutional denials of the legitimacy of same-sex attractions have to be faced the physical dangers to personal safety, threatened emotional connections to family, the condemnation of many religious organizations and the threat to employment and housing, all of which play out in a number of ways according to the individual's circumstances.

In addition to the efforts of society to control behavior based on gender, we must also consider that there are varying degrees of value placed on one's gender, regardless of whether behavior and appearance are consistent with expected gender roles. Males are more highly valued than females and wield more power and privilege because of their sex. To the extent that males do not *act like* males, they lose that power and privilege and are marginalized. To the extent that women live out their prescribed gender role they have less power and privilege. To the extent that women step out of their prescribed gender role they also lose power, privilege, and protection. Pharr (1988) argues that homophobia is a weapon of sexism. Simply put, the fear of being labeled gay, lesbian, or queer discourages men *and* women from stepping outside of their assigned gender roles. Calling a strong, outspoken woman "a dyke" is a way to silence her voice or at the very least to marginalize her message. One of the most frequently heard and most effective ways to keep boys and men in line with their gender roles is to call them "sissies," "fags," "ladies," or to tell them they "throw like a girl." At the point where gender and sexual orientation intersect, oppression takes different forms for males and females. Gay men and boys who "flaunt" their orientation are at high risk for physical assault. Lesbians may be seen as a less serious threat to social arrangements since women have less power in the first place. However, to the extent that they are seen as infringing on male power, living outside the expected realm of male protection, they become vulnerable to rape and other forms of physical assault. In addition, given the gender inequities in economic arrangements, lesbians, especially those with dependent children, are more vulnerable to poverty.

Working with queer groups brings some special challenges for group facilitators, queer or straight. First is the issue of sexual orientation. In the USA, we live in a homophobic, heterosexist society. The oppression is personal, political, and institutional. Non-queer people may be sympathetic to the struggles of queers; they may be knowledgeable about the issues faced by queers. Yet heterosexual privilege prevents them from having first-hand experience of being queer in a straight world. Queer facilitators also grew up in a homophobic, heterosexist society and have their own internalized oppression to deal with. In addition, it is easy to generalize one's own experience to others, ignoring the many ways there are to live a queer life, resulting in a lack of sensitivity to sexual orientations other than one's own. In particular, bi-sexuals and transpeople are often not seen as "real" queers because they do not identify themselves as gay or lesbian, resulting in their specific issues being minimized or ignored.

The next challenge is gender. The facilitator, regardless of sexual orientation, needs to have a working knowledge of gender power dynamics. In addition, he or she must be willing to suspend expectations based on gender stereotypes. Since gender-bending is frequently associated with queer identity, the facilitator must be willing to address his or her own discomfort with women who appear or sound masculine, and with men who appear or sound feminine, as well as with androgynous and transpeople.

Class, too, must be considered. As in any group of people, those with more money and standing have the advantage of using their resources to protect themselves in ways that others do not. By the same token, those with influence and standing may feel themselves at a disadvantage, having much more to lose if they are "outed." Working-class and poor queers may be more vulnerable to street violence and family rejection. In addition, single queer parents in need of welfare may be treated harshly by the welfare system, and they face the real threat of losing custody of their children. Gender and class overlap within the queer population in the same way as they do in the population at large. The income gap between men and women means that, on the whole, same-sex male couples are more likely to be better off financially than same-sex female couples. Class differences are often overlooked by group workers, leading to a lack of understanding of the real fears and difficulties which beset those they work with.

The racial and ethnic make-up of a group is also of significance. Different racial and ethnic populations see their queer members differently. Historically, Native Americans have honored and respected those among them whom they call "Two Spirit People" (Brown 1997). However as white European culture has gained hegemony, homophobia has gained ground in those communities. African American queers' existence has often been denied within their own community. To a people fighting for their own survival, the existence of black queer people has been seen as everything from an embarrassment to a betrayal (Lorde 1982). Among some cultural groups in which gender roles are particularly rigid, queer people simply have no place. The one common experience many queer people of color or minority culture seem to share is a sense of "homelessness." As one African American lesbian put it, "I never feel like I can be completely myself. When I am with lesbians I am an outsider because I am black. When I'm with black women I am an outsider because I'm gay. I feel like I don't have a place I can truly be at home" (quoted in DeLois 1993: 73).

In reality, any group is made up of members who cross the boundaries of sexual orientation, ethnicity, class, and gender, as well as of religion, age and degree of able-bodiedness. Group facilitators cannot be expected to have an intellectual or intuitive grasp of all the possible ways in which these classifications play themselves out in individual lives. However, an understanding that power and privilege are attached to individuals on the basis of these categories is necessary in order to attend sensitively to the experiences that group members raise. Ideally, the facilitator can suspend the assumption that he or she knows or understands what a group member's experience is, allowing the member to be the expert on his or her own life.

What follows is a composite of excerpts from a typical YouthPride support group. On this particular night, Michelle, a regular participant, has brought a friend who she introduces as Paul. I am relieved that I have a name with which to tag this new person as a male since his appearance is androgynous and because I realize how uncomfortable I am not knowing whether I am talking to a male or a female. Paul addresses the group.

Paul: Hi, I'm Paul, and Michelle told me about this group. I'm 17 and my parents kicked me out of their house a year ago. I bummed around a while and finally came to live around here because I heard there were people like me here and I thought it might be easier than staying in my home town. I've got a part-time job now, I'm studying to take my High School Equivalency test, and I'm living with a group of college students who had an extra room and were looking for a roommate. Things are really cool and I'm glad to be here.

Lisa (aged 16): Hey, Paul, I'm glad you found us too. I feel lucky that my parents have been pretty supportive of me. When I came out to them they were pretty shocked, and I think they still think this is a "phase" (laughter from the group) or an experiment, but mostly they have been OK.

Frank (aged 18): Man, my parents still don't even *know* about me. My old man would kill me, and then probably shoot himself. It got so much easier once I left home for college. Still, when I go home it's hard to remember who I'm supposed to be there and leave my real identity behind at school.

Paul: Well, for me, there wasn't much of a choice about them finding out, once I decided that I wanted to live my life the way I really feel inside. See, the thing is, well . . . (*he glances nervously around the circle*). They still think of me as Paula. To them, I am their *daughter*, not their *son*.

(*The group is quiet for a moment.*)

Susan (aged 17): Wow, that's really tough. It took a lot of guts for you to do that, Paul.

Wesley (aged 16): You mean you're not a real guy?

Michelle (aged 18): What's that supposed to mean, Wes? How many times have gay guys heard that? Are *you* not a "real" guy cuz you don't like to screw women?

Wesley: No, no, that's not what I meant . . . I mean . . . well, I don't know what I mean. I'm sorry, Paul, I didn't mean anything bad by it. I just don't understand—

Kate: It's an interesting question though, Wes. And I think it raises some stuff that we all have to deal with but maybe we don't talk about very much. What does it mean to be a "real" man or a "real" woman? Is it just about who we desire sexually? Is it about how we feel inside? Is it about how we are perceived by the way we look? I have the experience sometimes of looking at somebody and not being able to tell if they are male or female. And I have to admit, that makes me uncomfortable. Why is it so important to know if we're talking to a man or a woman?

Jessica (aged 17): I guess so we know if we can hit on them or not. (*Laughter from the group.*)

Wesley: No, really. I mean, that may be part of it, but it does seem important to know, cuz I guess we talk to guys and girls differently. Maybe we expect girls to be interested in something different from guys, so we talk to them about different things.

Jessica: Yeah, sure, but . . . well, we *know* that isn't true – that guys aren't interested in just "guy" things, and girls aren't interested in just "girl" things, especially here, I mean among g/l/b/t/q people. Look around. There's Mark over there knitting – isn't that supposed to be a "girl" thing? And, Susan, I'm assuming that black eye you have is from a hockey game, right? (*Susan grins and nods.*) And contact sports are supposed to be "guy" things. And, Mark, I've seen you done up in more make-up than I would *ever* wear! So why *do* we get all hung up about what's guy stuff and what's girl stuff?

Frank: Well, I don't think I *do* get hung up on it. I mean, I treat everybody the same, doesn't matter if they're male or female.

Paul: I'm not sure why it makes a difference, but it does. And the question you asked about what's a real man or a real woman . . . from my own experience I know it isn't about what equipment you're carrying. For me, my equipment doesn't match my feelings. I *feel* like a man . . . *inside*. And what's more, I like the way people treat me when they think I'm a man better than I liked the way they treated me when they thought I was a girl.

Michelle: How is it different?

Paul: Well, first, I feel safer as a man. I don't have to worry about being raped. I feel like people look at me and decide if I'm capable of doing a job based on if I really *can* do it or not. Like, what I mean is . . . I went to apply for a job working on the loading docks down on the waterfront. Nobody gave me any grief about if I could handle the job, they just gave me a chance, and when I proved I could, I was on the crew. If I had done that as a girl, they would have said, "Oh, I don't think a girl is strong enough to do this," or "You don't want to work with a bunch of rowdy men all day," stuff like that. Then, even if they gave me a chance I'd have to put up with crap from the crew, probably every day for a long time. *And* I make a lot more money than I would if I had to do a "girl" job.

Michelle: Well, that is just so unfair!

Mark (aged 19): Yeah, it is unfair. But guys have to be willing to stick up for themselves, be willing to fight if someone disses them. So we may be safe from rape, but not from other physical violence. *And* as *gay* men, we're even *more* likely to get beat up if we don't "act" like men.

Frank: I hear that!

Kate: Valid points all around. It makes me wonder what that's all about, though. I mean, what is it that's so threatening for people that they feel like they need to beat other people up when we don't "act" like the sex we're presumed to be?

Frank: I don't really know the answer, but I do know that my father really would kick the crap out of me if I told him I was gay. Ever since I was little all I've ever heard from him about gays is what fags they are, how they aren't real men, how it "ain't natural," and some of the stuff he and his army buddies did to the queers in his unit.

Lisa: That's just ignorance.

Frank (*shaking his head*): I don't think so. I think it's deeper than just *knowing* stuff. It's real deep inside him that real men play sports, hunt, drink, screw women and are always tough and ready to fight.

Mark: Yeah, my dad is the same way. He really *did* kick the crap out of me when he found out I was gay. I was so glad to get away from that house, I'll never go back. I do miss my mom, though.

Paul: Your mom was cool with it?

Mark: Maybe not exactly "cool," but she didn't fly off the handle. She was sad, mostly, I think, cuz she knew how other people would react and how hard it could be for me. But it didn't change her love for me. She just wants me to be happy.

Lisa: Geez, that really *is* different from my family. My parents seem to think it's just kind of this cute little "phase" I'm going through and that when I get older and meet a good man I will "snap out of it."

Susan: Yeah, for me it's like "Oh, you know Susan! She's just a tomboy, but she'll grow out of it." They don't get it, so sometimes it feels like the real me is just invisible to them.

Kate: Seems like many of you have been really invalidated by your families, by society. (*Nods of agreement all around.*) Well, listen, time is almost up, so how about if we start to wrap it up? It seems to me we've talked about a lot of stuff tonight and a lot of it has been about how tough it is to be us. And there's no doubt that is true. But I was also thinking how glad I am to be a lesbian and not having to live up to other people's expectations of who I should be. So maybe as we do checkout, people could say one thing that makes you glad to be gay – or however you identify yourself.

Susan: I'm glad to be gay because I just love women!

Mark: I'm glad to be gay just because it's who I am.

Paul: I'm glad to be trans because I feel like I can finally really be who I am.

Michelle: I'm glad to be gay because I think I've had to think about things straight kids don't have to think about. And it makes me more involved in working to change things. I like feeling like I have some power to make the world a better place.

Lisa: I don't think I feel that way yet, but I hope I will some day. In the meantime, I'm glad I'm gay because . . . I like exploring the different parts of who I am. And if this is just a phase, well, I hope it lasts a long, long time! (*Laughter.*)

Work with g/l/b/t groups illuminates the level at which gender is socially constructed as well as uncovering the depth to which most of us accept assumptions about the meaning of gender. It also raises questions about assumptions we might make concerning the gender composition of a group. In subsequent sessions of YouthPride, the individual identified in the previous vignette as Paul, requested that the group call him/her Paula. Rather than see this as a diagnosable condition, a facilitator with a sensitivity to sexual orientation would recognize the on-going development of Paul/Paula in claiming all of his/her identity. At the same time the gender composition of the group could be seen as changing over time, without adding or losing a single member!

As we saw in Chapter 2, building on the Boston University model of group development (Garland *et al.* 1965), Schiller (1995) added a gender dimension, expanding on feminist understandings of gender. DeLois and Cohen (2000) have suggested that the relational model may also be applicable to mixed-gender groups in cases where the facilitator holds a feminist worldview and overtly stresses the relational values of mutuality and community. The consideration of sexual orientation, while challenging the construction of gender, further suggests that a relational model may depend more on the relative power of group members as defined by membership in a variety of social categories, such as race, gender, sexual orientation, and class, as well as the perspective of the facilitator. Continuing work to analyse group dynamics and development through the lens of relative power and privilege may shed new light on conceptions of group development, moving both toward a more complete understanding of the complexity of the interactions of a variety of simultaneously held positions of privilege and oppression.

Finally, what is relevant for work with groups including diverse sexual orientation can also provide a different perspective for working with any group. Examining the construction of gender can lead to challenging assumptions and stereotypes about what it means to be male or female, helping group members expand their understanding of what it means to be fully human.

Note

1   The term "queer" is used throughout this chapter solely to denote the entire population of gay men, lesbians, bisexual, transgendered, and transsexual individuals.

References

Brown, L. (ed.) (1997) *Two-Spirit People: American Indian Lesbian Women and Gay Men*, New York: Haworth Press.

DeLois, K.A. (1993) "How women come to identify as lesbian: a grounded theory study," Unpublished doctoral dissertation, Seattle: University of Washington.

DeLois, K.A. and Cohen, M.B. (2000) "A queer idea: using group work principles to strengthen learning in a sexual minorities seminar," *Social Work With Groups*, 23, 3: 53–67.

Garland, J., Jones, H., and Kolodny, R. (1965) "A model for stages of development in social work groups," in Bernstein, S. (ed.) *Exploration in Group Work: Essays in Theory and Practice*, Boston, MA: Boston University School of Social Work.

Lorde, A. (1982) *Zami, a New Spelling of My Name*, Freedom, CA: Crossing Press.

Pharr, S. (1988) *Homophobia: A Weapon of Sexism*, Inverness, CA: Chadron Press.

Schiller, L.Y. (1995) "Stages of development in women's groups: a relational model," in Kurland, R. and Salmon, R. (eds) *Group Work Practice in a Troubled Society*, New York: Haworth Press.

Chapter 10

Women First

A self-directed group for women with and without learning disabilities[1] – our experiences 1990–99

The members of Women First

Our group believes that:
all people are equal quality human beings
but women are treated unequally and unfairly and
disabled women are treated especially poorly.

Our group further believes that
all women are equal quality
and share the same needs, wishes
and entitlements with one another
but some women in the group
have far less chance of ever having
equality of opportunity with other women.

Who are we and why did we set up our group?

We are a group of women with and without learning disabilities who are part of a bigger group called Advocacy In Action. This is a collective of people in a Midlands city in the UK who believe that disabled people have value and rights in society which are not recognized and who have promised to fight together until everyone gets the same value and rights.

The women of Advocacy In Action did not like

- the social, leisure, education, advisory and health services on offer to disabled women
- the fact that our experience told us that the 'disability services' were developed for white disabled men by white non-disabled men
- the way the men in Advocacy In Action wanted to do all the talking all the time and kept butting in and putting us down
- the behaviour of disabled and non-disabled men towards us, which was without respect. They felt they could touch us, and kiss and have sex with us when we didn't want to – even our brothers, uncles, grandpas, staff and male patients in institutions where some of us had lived
- the fact that the men of Advocacy In Action did not take our opinions seriously and did not treat us as equal quality

- being expected by the men in the group to make all the teas and coffees and do the running about after them, or even to look after them a bit sometimes and 'fuss them up'.

We wanted a place where all women who wanted to could be together without the men getting in the way.

Men were not the only problem, though. We did not like the way some 'women in charge' behaved towards disabled women and the bad power that was used in this relationship. So the place we wanted would have to be one where some women did not put other women down or boss them about or try to feel they were better than others. We wanted it to be somewhere where we could:

- feel safe and start to share experiences
- cry if we wanted to, or get angry, or tell secrets
- support one another
- get strong
- have a laugh and a joke
- be proud to be who we are and celebrate our differences
- share what we had in common as women and build something good together.

We decided to meet on Tuesday mornings in the side office at Princess House, Nottingham, where Advocacy In Action was based. We hung a notice on the door that said:

WOMEN'S GROUP – FOR WOMEN ONLY – KEEP OUT MEN!

Someone said it would be a good idea to hang garlic on the door too!

The men didn't like it one bit – what we did when we set up our group. They hung around outside; kept shouting in to ask us if they could make us cups of tea and coffee; got angry with all the women.

The women thought it was great to have a women's group and we all looked forward to Tuesday mornings more than any other time.

How did we set up our group and make rules?

We all decided together that we would make the group. It wasn't just one woman's decision, like a boss or a manager or a nurse, no! We all felt the wish to be together, because we wanted to and needed to, and that's how we decided to get things up and going.

We made a number of promises to one another about how the group would work. We said:

- Any woman could join the group and be there for one another (she did not have to be seen by others or see herself as disabled) but that we were all there for the rights and wishes of disabled women.

- As a women's group we were part of the wider Women's Movement and the things they fought for.
- As women, we wanted to welcome black women and those of other ethnicities, older women, young women and teenagers, women who used signs, sounds and noises, and some of us needed to find out about what it meant to be a lesbian because we didn't know about this.
- Professional and paid women could come to the group but they must leave their job titles outside and be there as women first.
- No woman could be there as an 'expert' on other women – we were only experts on ourselves.
- All women, whether or not they were seen as disabled, should share their experiences honestly – no 'observers', 'carers', 'note-takers' – everyone should open up their lives and hearts.
- No 'group leaders', 'facilitators' (that's jargon for bosses!), 'advisors', 'therapists' (that's jargon for controllers) or 'counsellors' – we wanted to advise and support one another and move forward in our own space and pace and choose the direction together.
- No woman was to put any other woman down even if we disagreed with one another – we had been put down enough by the people outside our group. We promised to build each other up sky high!

What problems did we have to deal with?

It was very difficult for some women to speak out and very difficult for others to shut up. We had to learn to share conversation: we asked another woman to speak before we did, noisy women partnered up with quieter women, we played the five bean game (where you start with five beans and give one up each time you speak, so no one has more than five turns), and we used picture language and signs to help women without words to join in.

Challenging each other was difficult for everyone. Some women took it personally and cried when they were challenged, for example about their attitudes to other people. Some said 'we disabled women shouldn't get picked on!' Others were a bit patronizing and felt it wasn't fair to challenge women they thought were more vulnerable than themselves. We learned that challenge was about giving respect and treating one another on a level; that not being challenged was like being patted on the head and not taken seriously – it might mean we weren't sufficiently valuable or important to disagree with. We also learnt to challenge the idea and not the person so that we did not say hurtful things.

We had problems over making sure all women were valued. Some group members were racist. Some felt sorry for women who 'couldn't walk or talk', others that 'grannies would slow us up!' We needed to learn that the things that put us down were our real barriers and that it was our own lack of self-value that made us want to downgrade other women. We did lots of work on labels, our own and other women's. We rubbished the bad labels – tore them up and threw them in the bin,

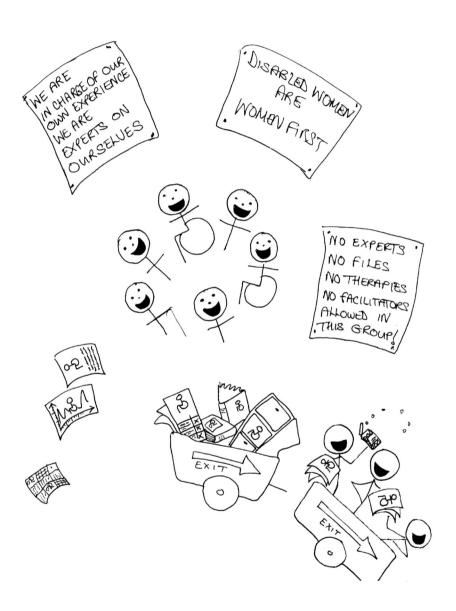

wheelchaired over them. We made lovely hearts full of compliments about ourselves and other women and put them on the wall. We listened to women's stories and learned about the other women's lives. We learned about different cultures and different experiences. We learned to feel proud to be disabled and proud to be ourselves – all shapes and sizes and colours. Women were proud of their wheelchairs and walking sticks – they put ribbons and stickers on them.

Some women had problems about saying 'no' to things they didn't want in the group and in their lives, and some women said that saying 'no' was about 'playing up'. Some women thought that it was not OK to get angry in case you got into trouble, like being put into the report book or sent to have a little word with the key worker. We needed to learn to get angry in the group – to trust in the strength of our feelings and our experiences. We realized that women weren't supposed to get angry, especially disabled women who were supposed to be grateful and suffer sweetly and play the saint. We went out to a local park and learned how to scream out loud, at the tops of our heads. We held hands and chanted 'NO-NO-NO'. We banged cushions down hard on the floor to get our tempers out and used the Empty Chair to tackle people who had hurt us. We used words, sign language, noises and sounds to tell the bad people where to get off.

Inequalities within the group

Working towards equality of opportunity meant first recognizing and owning our inequalities. This was hard because we wanted to be on a level. It felt much better to say 'Everyone is equal in here', but we knew in our hearts that it wasn't true and the way we behaved towards one another showed it up for a lie. So we had to take a long hard stare at ourselves and, yes, it was hard to look at what made us unequal but we wanted to try and do it.

Disabled and non-disabled women

Some non-disabled women tried to say, 'Well, we are all disabled one way or another, like wearing glasses or being the wrong shape'. Some women didn't want to say that they were disabled because they had learned to be ashamed of themselves and to try and hide their disabilities.

As a group we needed to accept our differences, to be proud of and celebrate them. But we also needed to look at how disability was to do with society not giving some women the same deal as others. We found out that the non-disabled women in the group had many more choices than the disabled women, like where to live, and who controlled their lives, and how they got around and about, and whether they could get jobs or partners or babies if they wanted them. We recognized the differences of power and privilege and agreed to work together to get more chances for the disabled women among us.

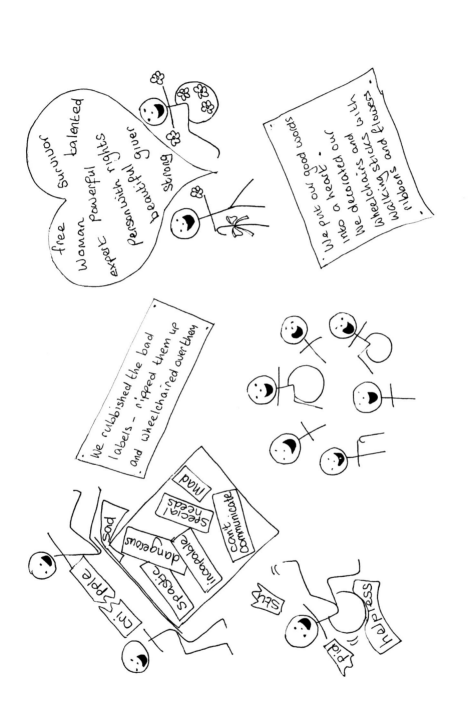

Paid and unpaid women

Some non-disabled and disabled women had jobs and some of them had paid jobs; other disabled and non-disabled women were not paid for the work they did in life. Some paid women wanted to say, 'Well, I'm here in my own time' or 'I'm not here as a professional' or 'I've got my volunteer's cap on today'. Some unpaid women said, 'I can't get pay for what I do 'cos I don't want my benefits cut off!' Other unpaid women said, 'I don't want to put a price-tag on the work I do'.

We found out there were big differences between paid and unpaid women, even where paid women were attending our group as volunteers. Women with good wages could come to the meetings in a warm jacket and trendy trainers, and run cars or afford bus-fares and taxi-fares, and buy a good lunch from the shop across the street. Unpaid or low-paid women like benefit-receivers could not make these choices so easily. Also, unpaid women found it harder to get their contribution to life recognized, recorded or rewarded and had more difficulties in seeing themselves or having others see them as effective and valuable workers and members of society. We recognized the differences of power and privilege and agreed to work together to get more chances and choices for paid work or higher benefits for the disabled women in our group and in society.

To address the power differences between paid and unpaid women, we worked within the group to value, record and reward everyone's contribution in terms of person-hours and the relative savings of not having used paid workers. No one got paid for being part of Women First. We chose also to work within our group in such a way that the value of the women who emptied the waste bins or stapled the hand-outs was of equal worth to us as the women who spoke out at conferences or went on protest meetings.

White women and black women

Our women's group had lots of racism in it. We had to learn what racism was and why it was bad for all women and all people but especially for those on the receiving end. We recognized why disabled people could become racist; if you were in an 'oppressed-down' group yourself, you learned how to 'press down' other people only too easily. We found out that to be black and disabled felt like a double burden when you were treated unfairly on both counts. So black disabled women were really up against it!

One woman said that a white male nurse called her 'Black Bess' and 'Sambo-Lil' because she was, he told her, his 'slave' while she was in hospital on a section. Another black woman wore her hat pulled low on her brow. Staff in her residential home had called her 'slap-head' and, feeling ashamed of her high ancestral fore-head, she had attempted to hide it. We also realized the racism towards Irish and Scottish women in our group and found out that, of all ethnic groups, these women had some of the worst lives of all in respect of their housing, benefits, health and life-expectancy.

We helped each other learn not to be racist. We made a rule:

NO RACISM IN OUR WOMEN'S GROUP – NOW OR EVER!

We were sad when one woman who wanted to stay racist chose to leave the group rather than stick to our rule.

We worked hard to make our group a welcoming place for women of all ethnicities and we enjoyed learning about other ways of life. We worked hard to attract women from different ethnic backgrounds to join us or support us. We celebrated the ethnic and cultural richness and differences within and among the group and our common humanity as women first. We recognized and owned the differences of power and privilege and agreed to work together to get more chances and choices for black disabled women and ethnically oppressed white disabled women within our group and in society.

Very young women, older women and women in between

When we looked at the age range in our group it was mostly between 25 and 55. This had something to do with educational services for younger disabled people being separate from adult provision such as day centres, and services for older people also cutting off at the other end. But we wanted to make sure that our group was an equal place for all ages and that it could truly meet the needs and represent the rights of all disabled women. We went into schools and colleges and helped young disabled women set up groups for themselves; we invited them to join our group or agree that we would stick together when we needed to. One young woman joined us at 18 to become one of our greatest speakers and teachers. We also made certain that older women knew they were welcome and would be made comfortable within the group. We had a strong voice from the over 60-year-olds amongst us.

We did not experience much age inequality within our group but we shared many stories of life outside and grew in our understanding of how very young and older disabled women were discriminated against in respect both of service provision and life in general. We recognized and owned the differences of power and privilege and agreed to work together to get more chances and choices for very young and older disabled women.

Care providers and care receivers

Some women could only get to come to the group if they had a 'carer' (care giver) with them. Often this was necessary, if they needed personal care or medication. But other times it felt more to do with the needs and insecurities of the carers!

Although every woman in our caring group was in reality a carer, for herself and for the women around her, there were big inequalities within the more formalized relationship of care-receiver and care-provider where members had carers in attendance. Women were often silenced by the presence of their carers or led to participate in a way that felt restrained or dishonest. This told the group lots about the power of carers, even where the carer said they hadn't got any power at all. It felt like women were a bit frightened of their carers, although many liked them as people. So we first said in the group:

* Carers should not be seen or heard.
* Personal care must be provided in private.

This meant that carers should bring their own activities to do in a separate room, rather than sit and listen in to what the group was doing, and that women should leave the group where possible to have their care needs met in private.

Women without their carers spoke out a 'very lot more'. They spoke out about not wanting to get on the wrong side of their carers or get things they'd said in the group reported back to their homes or day centres. One woman said she didn't want to make her carer sad. Disabled women all said that, when their carers were with them, the carer usually did all the talking and that was just the way it was. We decided to share some of these problems with the carers themselves and see what we could do to make things better.

The group told carers that if they would 'zip up' unless spoken to and let disabled women get a word in, and if they promised not to repeat things they heard in the group, and if they only spoke about their own feelings and experiences rather than as an 'expert' on the person they supported, then they would be welcome to take a more sharing part in the group. Some carers found it very difficult. Some tried hard, gave a great deal of themselves and got a lot out of the group. Other carers were told, 'Sorry! Keep staying outside 'til we need you!' Disabled women made the decisions about which carers belonged to the group and which didn't. It helped show them that they could take more control in relationships with the people serving their care requirements.

We recognized and owned the differences of power and privilege between 'carers' and people on the receiving end of 'care', and we agreed to work together to build a more equitable relationship within the care partnership both among group members and in the wider society.

Inequalities resulting from perceived levels of disablement

The group included:

* women with physical/learning/mental health disabilities
* women labelled as mildly/profoundly or multiply disabled
* walking women, crawling women and women wheelchair users
* women using words and women using noises, sounds or signs.

Perhaps the hardest inequalities to tackle within our group were those based around perceived levels of 'disablement'. The doctors and other professionals who took disabled people over and made them 'specialist territory' had split us into so many types and categories that we forgot what we had in common politically! This was ingrained into everyday language and showed itself in group put-downs such as: 'At least I'm not deaf and dumb like her!', 'Don't class me with that barmy lot', 'I feel sorry for her 'cos she's in a wheelchair', 'She's got special needs, she has, she can't do nothing for herself', 'Bless her! She can't talk', 'I'm deaf, not stupid!' The language told us that some disabled (and non-disabled) women felt embarrassed, intolerant, distanced or frightened by the disabilities of others and saw themselves as 'better-off', 'borderline', 'more able', 'higher grade', 'more intelligent'. Did this mean, then, that others were less valuable, with less right to be in the group, no point of view to voice or experiences worth sharing? Were some attributes, like intelligence or the ability to walk or mental 'stability', over-prized within the group? And, if this were true, what happened to women who could not demonstrate them?

To address these inequalities, we focused on what each woman in the group *could* do rather than what she couldn't do. We built up women's strengths and helped them practise the things they found difficult. Women with speaking differences or difficulties became front-line 'phone people within the group, or 'spoke' at meetings with pictures, signs and interpreters, because they had the right to and because in this way they could challenge non-disabled people's 'listening difficulties'. Women joined in by holding up papers and posters that their colleagues spoke to. Some very disabled women gave and got huge strength by just being there, at the front of whatever we were doing, proclaiming the right to witness and be witnessed, at all times, in all things.

We gave these messages loud and clear:

- We will not try to fit in, or apologise, or stay out of sight.
- We are not ashamed of ourselves.
- We have rights, not needs.
- We are strong proud women.
- And we are proud to be disabled.

We used pictures, videos, drama, signs and sounds, interpreters and objects of reference,[2] and we worked in the group to involve everyone fully. We built up a good language of power and possibility. We got rid of labels like 'non-walker' and 'non-talker' and replaced them with positive acclamations: 'wild wonderful women in wheelchairs' and 'women using noises, sounds and signs'. We exposed the label 'special needs' as a cover-up for 'second best'. We got rid of the special needs label and replaced it with the badge of 'unmet rights'.

We learned about the experiences of different women and challenged some silly ideas in the group around mental illness, blindness, deafness and profound learning disabilities. We stopped feeling sorry for women of different disability. We recognized the common experience of disability and started feeling angry together. We recognized and owned the politics and solidarity of disability and saw the vested interest in the professionals' 'divide and rule' approach. We agreed to work together to get more chances and choices for all disabled women, particularly those who usually got missed out because they were seen as 'incapable', 'dangerous' or 'sad'.

'Professional' and 'expert' opinion and personal experience

The final inequality we encountered within our group rested on the power of diagnostic labels. Women who had been labelled were in peril of being seen first and foremost in terms of the labels and, eventually, as seeing themselves solely along these negative parameters.

Our group welcomed women who had been excluded or assessed as 'inappropriate' for standard care provision because they were labelled as 'challenging'. Where the women wished to take part, the group worked towards unconditional acceptance based on mutual respect. This meant that no one judged anyone else's behaviour but also that behaviour which harmed or degraded wasn't tolerated. It took great time and love to help get rid of our bad labels and the underlying belief that 'other people know best about us'. We learned to challenge other people's opinions where they differed from our own and not to be intimidated by people in 'authority'. We replaced the diagnoses and the labels with glowing affirmations and worked hard to believe in all the good things we said about ourselves!

We worked hard to help every woman tell her own story in her own way, through words or signs or pictures, and to own the truth of her personal experience. Disabled women reclaimed feelings and lives. We learned to cry and mourn the things we had lost along the way and to build strong futures based on the expert testimony of our personal experience and our limitless potential.

Finally, we reclaimed one negative label and put it to good use. We were a group, we declared, who were all extremely proud to have 'challenging behaviour!'

What inequalities meant for Women First

Overall, the group's inequalities meant that, while some women could walk away from the issues or distance themselves from the feelings, others were caught in the traps of powerlessness, poverty and discrimination. They carried them into the group each session and took them out again when each meeting ended, and they lived in them between times. Women First worked hard towards equality inside and outside the group by recognizing what made us unequal and what changes we could effect.

Important statements and issues raised by disabled women within Women First

Messages to 'professionals' involved in the group

- You set the values and bring us in to get empowered.
- We do the hard work and you get the medals.
- We have the experiences, you do books about us.
- We stay poor, you get on.
- You have turned our experiences into something that belongs to you.
- You professional women use women's groups for your own agenda, then you say it was our idea and we wanted to do the things you want us to do, which we didn't always agree to or want to do.
- Some of our ideas get lost when too many outsiders get involved; professional people try to 'tame us down' or 'sweeten up smart' the things we say, or tell us not to make other people angry.
- In the end, you professionals got to toe the line with the people what pay you – that's why you aren't really part of Women First.

Messages to care providers

- The content of your plans and policies are about rights but the process or your plans and policies are about the denial of rights.
- Everyone is higher up the ladder than me – the doctor, house staff, social services, the driver on the bus to the day centre, the cook.
- Some women care providers exploit and rule over disabled women. They should act as women first rather than running on bad power.
- Some day care and residential staff are threatened by the group and pressurize or trick women into not attending. They change our timetables or hold review meetings to stop us coming here.
- Parents and carers (caregivers) don't always like what is happening when people grow stronger and become confident women and their own person. One 86-year-old mum said of her 50-year-old daughter: 'No girl of mine is going to cheek me and act naughty'. Another mother resented the loss of an unpaid companion and domestic help when her disabled daughter started to speak at conferences and, jealous of this freedom, persuaded her to give up. So parents and carers have a lot of power over women in our group.

Messages to society

- We disabled women aren't allowed to be sexual but then we also have to be fixed up with contraceptives and sterilization whether we want them or not. Disabled women get raped and abused by disabled and non-disabled people and no one bothers.

- Lots of our lives belong to other people. Natural events and processes, if you're disabled, get turned into 'specialisms' or 'expert territory' to be managed by people who know best.

Some things we learned and some things we did within ten years of Women First

- We learned how to involve women of many differing abilities in decision making within the group and we are proud of this.
- We linked in with and supported other women's groups, which was a good thing for disabled women to be able to do rather than just being supported all the time.
- We co-counselled each other on sexual and physical abuse – building on all the natural strengths, skills and qualities within the group and learning how to heal ourselves and one another.
- We 'sat on' material that professional women wanted to use to get famous and powerful which we felt belonged to us.
- We started to feel safe.
- We learned to enjoy taking risks.
- We represented ourselves and other women with learning disabilities at meetings, which was a first for Nottingham in 1990, and we consulted with many authorities and powerful groups to get our points heard and accepted.
- We discovered the tactics of confrontation.
- We learned to respect, value and enjoy ourselves and others within our relationships and partnerships and we built many new friendships. We reduced the barriers within the group through massage, body art, self-portraits, affirmations, gentle challenge and honest sharing.
- Women in power jobs outside the group promised to work with us to make things happen. Women allies chipped away inside the power strongholds while we bawled and battered on the outer doors.
- Our Women First group made a women's handbook about things we liked and didn't like in our lives – difficulties, problems, things we were proud of, our achievements and our goals, hopes and dreams.
- We helped plan and run the first national conference for women with learning disabilities which was about personal relationships.
- We took part in the *Betrayal of Trust* television documentary in 1991, which lifted the lid off the sexual abuse of people with learning disabilities.
- We helped other women's groups set up in Britain and overseas.
- We ran volunteer training for workers at the Nottingham Women's Centre and trained many women staff in local authorities and health authorities about issues for disabled women.
- We were one of the first women's groups for women with learning disabilities in Britain and we are proud of our achievements and proud of all the other women's groups that followed on.

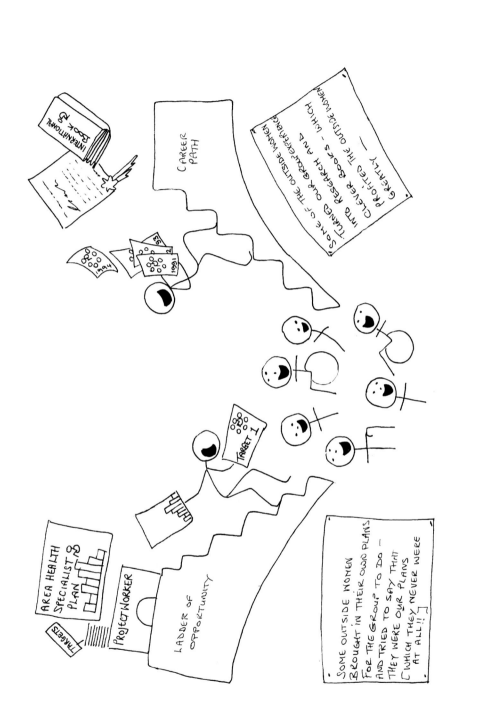

- We took no funding, charity or hand-outs – we ran on the money we earned by teaching and consultancy. We truly ran ourselves and were in full charge of everything we achieved, so no one could threaten us or shut us up!
- Our youngest member grew so greatly in confidence that she was able sometimes to leave her wheelchair at home and use a walking stick and public transport, which she never knew she could manage, while remaining proud of and powerful in her 'wheels' when she required them. Another woman confronted the brother who had abused her; others got married; many moved to first homes of their own.

As time went by

Women's groups eventually became 'flavour of the month' in the learning disability services world which was not always a good thing for learning disabled women. We heard stories of disabled women being 'placed in groups' or having 'women's group' put on their timetable, whether they wanted it or not.

When Advocacy In Action got big and famous, it started to happen to our women's group before we realized or could make sense of what was happening. All we knew was that the feeling changed and the group changed – we had to look hard at ourselves and ask 'Why are we here'? And who didn't want to be here in the first place but had got told to come and join in by someone else? So we put a stop to it, even though it meant the women leaving us who had not chosen to be in the group and who had been pleased to find out they had the choice to join or leave in the first place, which they didn't think they had!

And that's how we became Women First again – a small group in charge of ourselves and in charge of our lives. We carried on this way until eventually the group outlived its usefulness; women felt ready to move on and no longer needed its support.

Many still meet up these days as friends. Some went on to set up other groups and ventures, others moved out of touch. We know we can always re-form if we need to but, for the present, we are sustained by the strength which we drew from our time together and by the fact that, when we left the group behind, we took the goodness with us.

Notes

1   The term 'learning disabilities' is preferred here because 'disability' is a political term and its use denotes solidarity throughout the disabled people's movement, as opposed to the 'divide and rule' categorization by professionals between those with physical impairments, learning difficulties and mental health problems.

2   'Objects of reference' are an aid to communication, usually taking the form of a box of objects that can be pointed to or touched. For example, someone who is thirsty might indicate a cup. The objects can also be used in daily living so that, for example, someone without sight can feel fabric samples and indicate the kind of clothing they would like to wear that day.

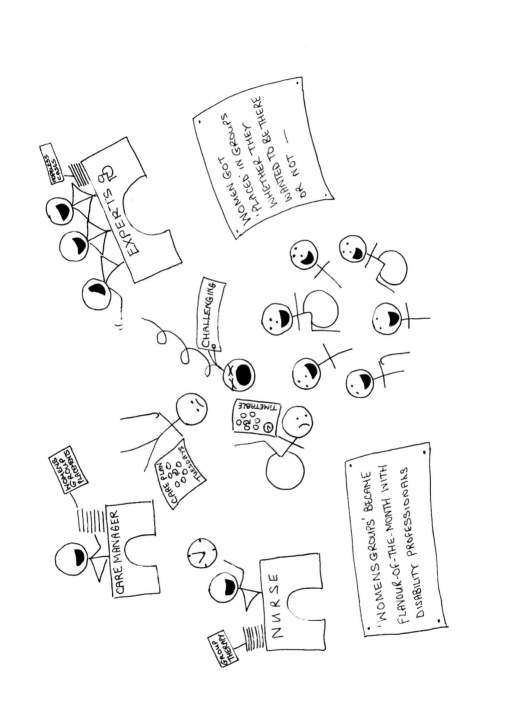

Chapter 11

Intersections of gender, race and ethnicity in groupwork

Edith A. Lewis and Lorraine M. Gutiérrez

Introduction

Understanding the importance of race, gender, and ethnicity in group work practice requires us to recognize and embrace the concept of intersectionality, the overlap and interaction of oppressions. Our lives illustrate the importance of inter-sectionality in unique ways. Race often dominates in decisions about group construction and group cohesion when the concern is heterosexual groups, for example. In the case of white women, the focus is often on gender as a primary criterion for consideration in group cohesion. We posit that the importance of intersectionality can be, and often is, overlooked in these situations. In the lives of women of color, there is no ability to separate the distinct contributions of race and/or gender, and the interaction of these social group memberships is more than either membership standing alone (Gutiérrez, L. and Lewis 1999).

Social group work that is empowering has cognizance of race, gender, and ethnicity. It is based on three premises:

- the importance of recognizing and incorporating the strengths of all members;
- that social group membership is a product of the strengths and activities of those who have preceded us; and
- that social workers can juggle the complexities of intersectionality as they engage in social group work practice.

In order to address all three of these premises, this chapter presents two examples of the ways in which group workers from two earlier decades engaged in practice that reflected the empowerment tradition in social work (Simon 1994). We have also included several exercises as "brain teasers" for social group workers gleaned from our discussions with workers attempting to employ those methods in their own work.[1]

The conceptual underpinnings of intersectionality

Brain teaser 1: Why make such fine distinctions? When designing "homogenous" groups, can we *not* assume that "women's groups" means feminist groups?

Heterogeneous groups by gender: roles of social group memberships and intersectionality

Our embracing of intersectionality as an organizing concept for group work is based on the historical underpinnings of the social work profession, social group work, and the work of feminist theorists of color during the last twenty years (Andulzua and Moraga 1983; Giddings 1984; hooks 1984; Davis 1996; Hill-Collins 1997; Gutiérrez, L. and Lewis 1999; Johnson 2001). The social ecological model has been central to this work. It is derived from the work of early settlement house workers and mutual support and aid groups operating in the nation's communities of color. The model is also used in more recent community development and community-building efforts such as those among migrant laborers in North Carolina and Village Health workers in Detroit, Michigan (Israel, *et al.* 1994; Gutiérrez, L. and Suarez 1999). In the model's conceptualization, participants and facilitators in group activities are not just individuals or simply members of families but are recognized also as members of communities and of the wider society. In recognizing this, we reach a more nuanced understanding of the role larger social systems play in working with and composing groups. Attention must be paid to these critical intervention points of "community."

Hurtado's work (1996) work illustrates the second, and perhaps more direct, influence on intersectionality. She focuses on the limited ability of some feminist writers to grasp the crucial role of intersectionality in moving beyond the dichotomous thinking so commonly found in the USA. Anthropologist and feminist scholar, Janet Hart (1996) is an example of someone who has moved beyond the dichotomous thinking of which feminists in the USA. are frequently accused (Hurtado 1996), to achieve this intersectionality. Hart has written about the women of the Greek Resistance, noting that due to the perceived similarities between their struggles and those of African Americans against racism the Greek women participating in her project were willing to speak candidly with her about their experiences. Hart's work exemplifies the ways in which a secondary construct (i.e. ethnicity) combines with the primary construct (gender) under study to form a wider lens and a greater ability to build cohesiveness in a group. This new lens can be used to inform group designs, processes, and outcomes.

In earlier work, we have outlined how our nation's insistence on a "melting pot" approach to interactions among the populace has marginalized some groups within the wider society. We termed those marginalized statuses *vis-à-vis* the wider society "social group memberships" (Gutiérrez, L. and Lewis 1994). In contemporary US society, those social group memberships include the "protected classes" recognized in the Constitution: *race, gender, class, religion*, and *national origin/ethnicity*. In addition, the societal marginalization of people due to *sexual orientation, physical and mental ability*, and *age* has earned their inclusion in this construct by most scholars in the field (Lewis 1989). Originally the scholarship on social group memberships focused on single social group memberships such as race or gender (Devore and Schlesinger 1987), and challenged research and scholarship in social work to consider them in analyses and reporting (Jackson *et al.* 1982; Green 1995; Lum 1996). These writers then set the stage for more recent research and scholarship on how these single memberships interact with one another to form a larger and more complex, not just additive, group work construct (Gutiérrez, L. *et al.* 1998; Spencer *et al.* 2000).

Social group memberships and intersectionality

Brain teaser 2: Provide working definitions for these single social group memberships, including how they are marginalized in your society, and for any existing groups you are aware of that serve them:

- mental and physical disabilities, visible or hidden
- age
- gender
- ethnicity
- race
- mental health
- sexual orientation
- socio-economic status.

It should be noted that all of these single social group membership statuses may be determined along a continuum. In other words, one's status as a transgendered individual is not dichotomous. It is not that one is *either* transgendered *or* not. Instead, one can conceive of transgendered persons of color who are active in what might be considered vastly dissimilar gendered group activities during their lifetimes. For example, a women's group with which one of the authors is associated gave a "Welcome to the Sisterhood" party for a transgendered individual who was also a person of color and had chosen to adopt a simple life with very limited income.

Understanding intersectionality from the standpoint of social work practice in general

Brain Teaser 3: The world is already too complex. Isn't it useful to focus on a single social group membership when forming a group and simply acknowledge the potential impact of others?

One of the maxims of social work practice is "Start where the client is." In our design and formation of groups, social work practitioners may also construct a group for one purpose when its actual benefit might be in an entirely different arena. How many women's groups have been started in agencies across the USA whose work broadens immediately into issues of economic status, age, or race? Both of us have been involved in group activities that had been begun by practitioners for one purpose, when the actual needs of the group members reflected an altogether different social group membership (Gutiérrez, L. and Lewis 1994). Flexibility and critical reflection are warranted throughout the group process so that groups may benefit from these "alternative routes."

One example of this was a series of training groups for seasoned social work practitioners on issues of race and ethnicity as social group memberships. The trainers had contracted with a state agency to provide these group-based programs in various district agencies over a period of two years, and had been able to develop a "script" from which to work together. Entering one site approximately eighteen months after beginning to work together, the trainers began their script only to find the group participants shifting the focus of the discussion to issues of sexual orientation. After three attempts to move the program back to a singular discussion of race, the trainers decided to stop, report to group members their perceptions about group interactions and areas of tension, and then ask about their percep- tions about the nature of the shift. It appeared that this particular area of the state was a hotbed of homophobia and heterosexism, and that gay/lesbian/bisexual professionals felt unsupported by those "womens'" and "people of color" organi- zations they had attempted to engage in their struggle. They then demonstrated, as had the majority of participants at that particular workshop, an operational knowledge of all of the materials contained in the original "script" planned for the groups. With that information, and with the agreement of all parties involved, the group moved into a discussion of how the intersectionality of sexual orientation, race and gender might influence the ability of these professionals to work together. Honest discussions about feelings of "betrayal," "needing to focus on the most important problem," and "how to get district to do the right thing" then ensued. The purpose of the work group shifted from education to one requiring skills in conflict management and organizational/community change.

Beginning where group members were, and having frank and open discussions as a part of group formation and process, helped the entire group move consciously through the permutations of their relevant social group memberships. Being aware of ways in which certain portions of groups exhibit behaviors associated with particular social group memberships and having the ability to address areas of conflict are critical for social group workers.

What has all of this to do with group process and construction?

While many of our colleagues continue to struggle with single social group memberships' impact on groups, we challenge those who have had the opportunity to work more comfortably with these single memberships to move beyond them and incorporate intersectionality into their work. As a result of this shift, a number of new questions are raised about group construction, preparation, and process.

> *Brain teaser 4*: Some questions to ponder on intersectionality:
>
> • When beginning to think about the multiple social group memberships represented in any group enterprise, and particularly in an empowerment-oriented group, is it wise to address a number of questions/issues in the formation period of the group?
> • If empowerment is a useful construct cross-culturally, do we need to change the language/terminology/presentation to engage further all cultures represented in the group project?
> • How do we use standard group strategies, such as role-play, teams, co-facilitation, and feedback, while also recognizing the importance of intersectionality?

The social group work method as a process requires being realistic about what can and cannot be done. The conflicts between different social groups in our society did not begin overnight and will not be resolved within a single group meeting. What is required in empowering social group work is reflexivity about the conflicts inherent in women's lives. As exemplified in the social ecological model, when one membership is being advantaged, another may be potentially disadvantaged (Germain 1973). In the case of group members whose intersectionality has relied on these interactive memberships, the requirement to focus on one to the exclusion of the other can be internally disconcerting. The "splitting" required, in some cases, is just not possible in a multiple-social-group-integrated person. Thus, when women are asked to divide themselves on the basis of race, increasingly we are finding that bi-racial women wish to be recognized as belonging to more than one category, even if that category is "person of color." Instead, Jordan's "person in relationship" model (Jordan 1997) may be the most useful in highlighting for group facilitators and members the ways in which complex interactions with one's family, group, community, and society might be negotiated. This complexity in group work can be achieved by group facilitators being deliberate in the formation of groups, identifying their goals and objectives, and addressing specific differences and finding similarities in the group (Gutiérrez, L. and Lewis 1999).

Learning from our pasts: all of our ancestors have brought us to this place

Brain Teaser 5: In managing conflict between staff and service consumer statuses – how can we support both consumers' and staff's agency?

Race, ethnicity, and gender have been essential elements of social group work since its inception. Although the early group workers did not use our contemporary language or concepts, their theories and practice have much to offer us. In addition, recognizing the hard-won lessons of early group workers of color can be informative. We present descriptions from two group programs serving US residents of color in the twentieth century that can teach us about group practice today.

From youth leadership to a movement: the Mexican American Movement

Scholarship on Mexican American/Chicano activism is typically regarded as having begun in the post-Second World War era. This view of our history overlooks the significant work of other organizations such as the Mexican American Movement (MAM) and of early labor struggles in bringing Mexican Americans together to question their social conditions (Gutiérrez, F. 1984; Muñoz 1989).[2]

Mexican American historians now identify the MAM as one of the first campus and community-based organizations developed to advocate for the status of Mexican Americans in California and the southwest (Muñoz 1989; Sanchez 1993). However, these histories have not fully recognized the crucial role that social group work played in organizing and supporting these efforts. The story of the organization of the MAM provides an example of culturally appropriate ways in which intersectional social group work programs can contribute to social action.

The MAM was an outgrowth of the Mexican Youth Conference organized by the YMCA in Los Angeles in 1934 (Gutiérrez, F. 1984; Muñoz 1989). The YMCA became involved in this work when it received a grant to hire Tom Garcîa, a Mexican American group worker, to create a youth leadership program in order to reduce "juvenile delinquency" in the city. The focus of the youth program was to use group work methods to engage young men in developing "character, good citizenship, and desirable values" (Muñoz 1989). The program included an annual weekend conference where young men who had been selected for their leadership potential met and engaged in educational workshops and sports activities (Sanchez 1993). One goal of these annual conferences was to develop local and regional groups for Mexican American youth (Gutiérrez, F. 1984).

The Mexican Youth Conference reached out to youth organizations in the region and, with increasing autonomy, began publishing its own magazine, *The Mexican Voice*.

The Mexican Voice, edited by Félix J. Gutiérrez, began as a mimeographed sheet, but, by 1941, was typeset with original Mexican themed art on the covers

(Gutiérrez, F. 1984). Topics covered by the magazine included the social conditions of Mexican Americans, news of local and regional clubs, profiles of successful Mexican Americans, sports news, and editorials on current events. The magazine was an effective organizing tool which brought new members and groups together. Although the focus of the YMCA had been on young men, many of the contributors of and subscribers to this new magazine were young women.

Organizing activities undertaken by members of the Mexican Youth Conference led to the development of the Girls' Conference in 1941. Dora Ibañez, the sister of an active member of the Mexican Youth Conference, initiated the Girls' Conference. One motivation for a separate conference for girls was the concern of many Mexican American parents that their daughters should not attend a weekend retreat with single young men. The content of the Girls' Conference paralleled the program held for boys, and many joint banquets and other activities took place. As an organization for young women, the Girls' Conference also included gender-specific topics such as gaining support for higher education for women, conflicts with parents regarding gender-appropriate behavior and the role of women as community leaders (Moreno 1939). Its creation reflected the intersection of gender and ethnicity for these young women and a desire to address the specific challenges they faced (Gutiérrez, F. 1984).

In 1942, the leadership of the Mexican Youth Conference voted to leave the auspices of the YMCA to incorporate as an independent non-profit organization called the Mexican American Movement (MAM).The goals of the MAM incorporated many of the values of the YMCA group workers, such as community, self-education, and democracy, in addition to broader goals emphasizing the importance of improving the conditions of the Mexican American community and so reflecting an awareness of the intersectionality of ethnicity, gender and class.

The Mexican Youth Conference and the MAM were actively involved in group programs for young Mexican American men and women from 1934–50. Although the MAM was relatively short-lived, it contributed to the development of the community and its members in many ways. Connecting and bringing together Mexican American young men and women from Arizona and California through its youth conferences and publications contributed to the solidarity of this population. The dialogue that took place also contributed to the consciousness and awareness of the conditions of Mexican Americans in the region. Equally important was the way in which these group work programs enhanced the leadership skills and social development of the participants in the conferences and in the MAM (Muñoz 1989; Sanchez 1993). Many of the participants went on to become educators, group workers, and attorneys in the greater Los Angeles area, and used the skills they had developed to create new organizations such as the Association of Mexican American Teachers (Gutiérrez, F. 1984; Muñoz 1989).

The historical example of the Mexican Youth Conference and the MAM provides insights for current ethnically appropriate and gendered group work. Although the leaders of the YMCA were primarily white and Protestant, they strategically chose a Mexican American group worker to create the initial Mexican Youth Conferences.

This reinforces the importance of hiring and working with those who have an intimate familiarity with the community. The cultural knowledge of this group worker led him to make strategic decisions in how the group was formed. The organization's encouragement of *The Mexican Voice*, the Girls' Conference, and other autonomous activities, is a demonstration of the ways in which group workers who are conscious of intersecting identities can support group and community development activities that may go beyond the initial plan.

The Wilder Foundation Community Group Project for Ex-Offenders

In 1971, one of the authors, Edith Lewis, was working in a residential program for men and women completing prison sentences and preparing to re-enter their communities. This demonstration project, funded by the Wilder Foundation, used a group format for the majority of its work, and only in rare instances would individual or family counseling take the place of the group as the primary intervention tool.

The Wilder Community Group Project for Ex-Offenders was an innovative program in many respects. Some social work scholars have argued that we experience cyclical periods of support for those who utilize traditional social work services, with more or less support available depending upon the "novelty" of the group (Lewis 1989; Jansson 1994; Gutiérrez, L. and Lewis 1999). In 1970, we knew very little about male ex-offenders and their families. We knew even less about women who had been incarcerated, particularly women of color. The relationships between women's incarceration and previous substance misuse, child sexual and or physical abuse and neglect were largely undocumented at that time. Even the now-recognized and employed standards for social group work (Rose 1989; Garvin and Reed 1995) had not been systematically taught in social work programs. The Wilder Community Group Project for Ex-Offenders added a great deal to our knowledge base about the types of intervention for ex-offenders that would limit if not eliminate their recidivism. The early groups in that project also taught us a great deal about heterogeneity versus homogeneity within groups, and about group size and managing conflict. Some illustrations of these lessons follow.

The body of staff chosen to work with individuals who were leaving the corrections institutions in the state of Minnesota but not yet released from the Department of Corrections was eclectic in background and training. Two were Adlerian psychologists, four were MSW practitioners, four were undergraduate or graduate social work practice students from area institutions who had an academic concentration in group work, and six were formerly incarcerated individuals who had developed a strong commitment to smoothing the transition for those who would follow them. The staff met twice-weekly as a group and literally taught one another the group skills each had learned in their respective disciplines, supplementing, in the case of the social work interns, the social group work literature. All members were challenged weekly to think about how these principles from the various disciplines influenced their actual work in the groups they co-facilitated each day. The goal was to take a strengths' perspective with the program participants, building on their experiences of self-efficacy rather than simply pathology.

As a result of being in this practice environment, Edith Lewis learned that gender, race and ethnicity significantly influence interactions within a group setting. As the group project continued, men's and women's groups began to be substituted for mixed groups. She also learned that group size had a great deal to do with group outcomes, and so lobbied to change the size of groups from more than twenty-five per session to fewer than fifteen (it was not until much later that standard practice became eight to twelve group members in therapeutic and task groups). Most importantly, the use of co-facilitation as a way of enhancing group outcomes grew out of this experience as the staff learned that they could work together in ways that would foster rather than thwart discussion in both homogeneous and hetero- geneous groups. As a result, the staff began to focus on their own permutations and multiple social group memberships/interactions so that they could work more effectively, for example, with ex-offenders who had a history of violence against women and had earlier scapegoated women co-leaders (see Blacklock, Chapter 6, this volume), those who were coming home to the responsibilities of partners and children, and those women who wished to avoid re-incarceration but who had limited educational backgrounds and economic resources.

Another set of practices engaged in by the Wilder staff was setting a specific time limit for each group, strengthening group cohesion rather than having open membership, doing initial screening of members for their fit with a group-oriented program, encouraging group members to tell their own stories, checking in with their co-facilitator to pre-plan the group's activities, and meeting at the end of the session to debrief one another. Remnants of these group work strategies can be disaggregated from current group work research with women. In one study of a psychosocial group for women offenders, for instance, Pomeroy et al. (1999) incorporated the training of group co-facilitators, a time-limited model, and the gender make-up of the group participants. Smokowski et al. (1999) and McQuaide and Ehrenreich (1998) recognize the impact of leader intersectionality on group dynamics, one of the reasons for group co-facilitation and post-group debriefing. Attention to group size and duration is key to the findings of McKay et al. (1999) regarding urban multiple family groups with children exhibiting inappropriate behaviors. Parsons' findings (2001) continue to support the importance of attention to group composition for group outcomes.

Some final considerations for social group work

> *Brain Teaser 6*: Have the social sciences responded to the call
> simultaneously to address race, gender, sexuality, age, disability and class?
> What direction should social group work with women of color take, given
> the challenges of intersectionality?

As outlined in earlier portions of this chapter, some studies still ignore the inter-sections of various social group memberships and some are wrestling with them. We can see, however, that progress has been made in placing people back within their environments based on their experience, rather than shaping them to our conceptual perspectives on how individuals in groups interact. Our critique is that many of our conceptual frameworks are limited because those perspectives, at best, incorporate single group memberships. It is through using the types of strategy described in the MAM and Wilder Foundation projects that social work practitioners can further inform the profession. These include building co-leadership reflective of the interesectionality inherent in the heterogeneous group and recognizing that intersectionality by addressing both gender and other memberships such as class and ethnicity. In addition, intersectionality leads us to recognize that group programs are themselves social constructs, changing with the historical, social, and political contexts they operate within.

During the last thirty years, social group workers have added complexity to the understanding of gender with the recognition of intersectionality. It is impossible to discuss gender without also discussing the various challenges to our use of the dichotomous variable of gender (see Chapter 9, by Kate DeLois, this volume). We can no longer design and operate groups under the notion that one has either one gender or the other. Instead, we are now increasingly forced to ask potential group participants "How do you define gender and what importance does it have in your life today?" Furthermore, there is difference and diversity within gender, in relation to ethnicity, sexuality, (dis)ability, age, socio-economic class, and so on. Practice that does not recognize this keeps group members from obtaining full benefit from the group. The history of how organizations for people of color have become spontaneously gendered, while developing more complex permutations along intersectional lines, challenges contemporary practice. The "road to inter-sectionality" is paved with such challenges and lessons. We suggest that we can build upon those lessons from the past to address the needs of those who work in groups, now and in the future.

Notes

We appreciate the assistance we received from Félix Gutiérrez and the editors of this book in developing this chapter.

1   We are grateful to the staff of the Office of Student Services at the University of Michigan for their contributions to the 'Brain teasers' used in this chapter.
2   Lorraine Gutiérrez has an intimate sense of this heritage, as her parents were among the organizers of the MAM in the 1930s.

References

Andulzua, G. and Moraga, C. (eds) (1983) *This Bridge Called My Back: Writings by Radical Women of Color*, New York: Kitchen Table, Women of Color Press.
Davis, A. (1996) "Gender, class and multiculturalism: rethinking 'race' politics," in

Gordon, A. and Newfield, C.C. (eds) *Mapping Multiculturalism*, Minneapolis: University of Minnesota Press.

Devore, W. and Schlesinger, E. (1987) *Ethnic-Sensitive Social Work Practice*, St Louis, MO: Mosby.

Garvin, C. and Reed, B. (1995) "Sources and visions for feminist social work: reflective processes, social justice, diversity, and connection," in van Den Bergh, N. (ed.) *Feminist Practice in the 21st Century*, Washington, DC: NASW Press.

Germain, C. (1973) "An ecological perspective in casework practice," *Social Casework*, 54, 7: 323–330.

Giddings, P. (1984) *When and Where I Enter: The Impact of Black Women on Race and Sex in America*, New York: Morrow.

Green, J. (1995) *Cultural Awareness in the Human Services*, 2nd edn, Needham.

Gutiérrez, F.F. (1984) "Mexican-American youth and their media: *The Mexican Voice*, 1938–1945," Paper presented at the Annual Meeting of the Organization of American Historians, Los Angeles, CA, USA.

Gutiérrez, L. and Lewis, E. (1994) "Community organizing with women of color: a feminist approach," *Journal of Community Practice* 1, 2: 23–44.

—— (1999) *Empowering Women of Color*, New York: Columbia University Press.

L. Gutiérrez, Parsons, R., and Cox, E. (1998) *Empowerment in Social Work Practice: A Sourcebook*. Pacific Grove, CA: Brooks/Cole.

Gutiérrez, L. and Suarez, Z. (1999) "Empowering Latinas," in Gutiérrez, L. and Lewis, E. (eds) *Empowering Women of Color*, New York: Columbia University Press.

Hart, J. (1996) *New Voices in the Nation: Women and the Greek Resistance, 1941–1964*, Ithaca, NY: Cornell University Press.

Hill-Collins, P. (1997) "Women in families: race, gender and class," Keynote speech at the Annual Meeting of the National Council on Family Relations, Chicago, IL.

hooks, b. (1984) *Feminist Practice: From Margin to Center*, Boston, MA: South End Press.

Hurtado, A. (1996) *The Color of Privilege: Three Blasphemies on Race and Feminism*, Ann Arbor: University of Michigan Press.

Israel, B., Checkoway, B., Schulz, A., and Zimmerman, M. (1994) "Health education and community empowerment: conceptualizing and measuring perceptions of individual, organization and community control," *Health Education Quarterly*, 21, 2: 149–70.

Jackson, J.S., Tucker, M.B., and Bowman, P.J. (1982) "Conceptual and methodological problems in survey research on black Americans", in Lui, W.T. (ed.) *Methodological Problems in Minority Research*, Chicago IL: Pacific–Asian American Mental Health Research Center.

Jansson, Bruce (1994) *The Reluctant Welfare State*, Pacific Grove, CA: Brooks/Cole.

Johnson, R.B. (2001) "Coalition politics: turning the century," in Andersen, M.L. and Hill-Collins, P. (eds) *Race, Class and Gender: An Anthology*, Belmont, CA: Wadsworth/ Thomson Learning.

Jordan, J.V. (ed.) (1997) *Women's Growth in Diversity: More Writings from the Stone Center*, New York: Guilford.

Lewis, E. (1989) "Role strain in African American women: the efficacy of support networks," *Journal of Black Studies*, 20, 2: 155–69.

Lum, D. (1996) *Social Work Practice and People of Color*, Pacific Grove, CA: Brooks/Cole.

McKay, M.M., Gonzales, J., Quintana, E., Kim, L., and Abdul-Adil, J. (1999) "Multiple family groups: an alternative for reducing disruptive behavioral difficulties in urban children," *Research in Social Work Practice*, 9, 5: 593–607.

McQuaide, S. and Ehrenreich, J. (1998) "Women in prison: approaches to understanding the lives of a forgotten population," *Affilia*, 13, 2: 233–46.

Moreno, S. (1939) "First organizational meeting – Mexican Girls' Conference", *The Mexican Voice*, Spring: 5.

Muñoz, C. (1989) *Youth, Identity, Power: The Chicano Movement*, London: Verso Press.

Parsons, R. (2001) "Specific practice strategies for empowerment-based practice with women: a study of two groups," *Affilia*, 16, 2: 159–79.

Pomeroy, E.C., Kiam, R., and Abel, E. (1999) "The effectiveness of a psychoeducational group for HIV-infected/affected incarcerated women," *Research in Social Work Practice*, 9, 2: 171–87.

Rose, S. (1989) *Working with Adults in Groups: Integrating Cognitive Behavioral and Small Group Strategies*, San Francisco CA: Jossey-Bass.

Sanchez, G. (1993) *Becoming Mexican American: Ethnicity, Culture and Identity in Chicano Los Angeles, 1900–1945*, New York: Oxford University Press.

Simon, B.L. (1994) *The Empowerment Tradition in American Social Work*, New York: Columbia University Press.

Smokowski, P.R., Rose, S., Todar, K., and Reardon, K. (1999) "Postgroup-casualty status, group events and leader behavior: an early look into the dynamics of damaging group experiences", *Research in Social Work Practice*, 9, 5: 555–74.

Spencer, M., Lewis, E. and Gutiérrez, L. (2000) "Multi-cultural perspectives on direct practice in social work," in Allen-Meares, P. and Garvin, C. (eds) *Handbook of Direct Practice in Social Work: Future Directions*, Thousand Oaks, CA: Sage.

Chapter 12

From support to empowerment

Caregiver connections

Betsey Gray and Tara C. Healy

In the USA, the care of frail elders primarily involves women as care receivers and as caregivers. Most frail elders (80 percent) in need of assistance are cared for in the community (Office of Management and Budget Watch 1990). Women live longer and experience a greater degree of disability and poverty as seniors than do men (Siegel 1993). Almost 90 percent of the care received by frail elders living in the community is provided by women who are not paid for their labor (Briar and Kaplan 1990). These caregiving women average 57 years of age; 25 percent are between the ages of 65 and 75, and 10 percent are over 75 years. More than half this population of caregivers reports incomes in the low–middle range and 31 percent have incomes below the poverty line. It is also important to realize that one-third of the caregivers rate their own health as poor (Bunting 1989: 65). The estimated costs of the provision of unpaid caregiving labor was $196 billion in 1997, an amount exceeding what was spent on nursing home and paid home health care combined (Arno *et al.* 1999). The physical, emotional, social, and economic burdens of providing this care can be enormous. Even the formal care providers for frail elders are primarily women, including many women of color, who are paid very poorly for their work (Collopy *et al.* 1990). Although issues of gender are central to caregiving, relatively little attention has been paid to how gender influences group work with caregivers.

Caring as women's work

Caring is central to the experience of women (Scheyett 1990). Caring has been defined as the "mental, emotional, and physical effort involved in looking after, responding to, and supporting others" (Baines *et al.* 1991: 11). The social construction of gender cannot be separated from the social construction of caring as women's work involving the oppression of "compulsory altruism" (Baines *et al.* 1992: 22). Caring involves both caring *about* another and caring *for* another (Ungerson 1983). Caring *for* typically involves physical labor, and caring *about* involves emotional labor. Women have all heard disparaging remarks about other women who are assumed not to care about a loved one when faced with difficulty in providing care for that person (Baines *et al.* 1991). Because the ethic of care (see Baines *et al.* 1992) is a deeply ingrained value that is the foundation of ethical deliberation for women (Gilligan 1983), and is also associated with women's sense of self-worth (Miller 1977), moral pain often arises when women are faced with difficult choices due to the scant resources for care provided by society.

Empowerment approaches include consciousness-raising about beliefs that are oppressive (Cox and Parsons 1994). Given the "compulsory altruism" embedded in beliefs about the gendered responsibility for caregiving in our society, group work with caregivers must include consciousness-raising about gender if it is to empower women. The ethical dimensions of decisions about caregiving within families require consciousness of the gendered values intertwined with those decision-making processes. To ignore the moral pain of women caregivers is to ignore the heart of the gendered dilemmas they face. Thus consciousness-raising must also involve highlighting the relationship between gendered values and the experience of guilt and shame.

This chapter considers ways in which gender affects process in caregiver groups and the ways that the social construction of gender influences perceived choices experienced by women who are caregivers. We begin by contrasting traditional and feminist models of group development. We then illustrate practice implications by describing an all-women group and a mixed-gender group. Gendered issues relating to the moral dimensions of decision making in families are addressed. Finally, we suggest ways to move from support to empowerment in caregiver groups by focusing on often neglected issues of gender.

Group development

As our society ages, more attention is being placed on the role of the caregiver and ways to meet caregivers' needs. It is evident that stress and isolation often characterize the lives of those caring for an elderly person. Toseland (1995) identifies caregiver groups as an effective intervention for reducing these symptoms. As stated earlier, the care of elders in our society is a role primarily assumed by women. It is therefore not surprising that caregiver groups are composed mostly of women.

Historically, group development has been classified according to stages. Most models identify groups as going through three to five stages. Traditional models (Garland *et al.* 1965) include such stages as the following:

1   pre-affiliation
2   power and control
3   intimacy
4   differentiation and
5   separation.

In contrast, Schiller's (1997) relational model of group development, grounded in feminist theory, sees women as more likely than men to establish a relational base before challenging each other (see Chapter 2, this volume, for a detailed account of this model).

Our contention is that the lessons learned from women in support of Schiller's model are applicable for caregiver groups, including those with male members. Issues faced by men and women who are caregivers are gendered and, because the members of caregiver groups are predominantly women, we propose that facilitators of these groups adopt the relational model as a guide for all caregiver groups. The following is a brief description of the contrast between the middle stages in these models of group development.

The second stage of group development in the traditional model is the "power and control" stage in contrast with the "developing a relational base" stage of Schiller's model. In this stage, traditionally, members are expected to challenge the facilitator and other members. Conflict is expected to emerge among members, and between members and the facilitator. In contrast, members are seen to develop a sense of safety in the relational base stage of Schiller's model. The depth of connectedness developed in the stage of mutuality and interpersonal empathy sets the stage for challenge and change in Schiller's model. The practice examples below suggest that the relational model has greater applicability to caregiver groups (with their predominantly female membership) than do more traditional models.

Practice examples

The following examples of caregiver groups are discussed in relation to our recommendations for facilitators of caregiver groups.

Group A: an all-women caregiver group – Mary's experience

Mary was a 65-year-old member of an all-women group. At the first meeting, she shared her story of caring for both her mother and mother-in-law. She said that she had had to quit her job and remain at home with them. Her husband provided some support but, essentially, all the caregiving was done by Mary. Mary said that she was feeling very isolated and had no time to spend with her husband, family or friends. She and her husband had been invited away for the weekend but her mother-in-law had "made it clear" that she would not stay with anyone but Mary. In addition, Mary said that she "could never leave them. I would feel so guilty if something happened." The only times that Mary ventured out of the house were when her husband could stay with the two older women.

Group B: a mixed-gender caregiver group with one male member – Philip's experiences

Philip was a 60-year-old man caring for his wife who was chronically ill. Philip was the only male member of this group. In the first meeting of the group, members shared their stories and purpose for attending group. Philip quickly became the most vocal about his situation and spoke of the frustration of caring for his wife. He confronted several women early on about issues related to caregiving. Over the next several meetings, Philip became increasingly angry when he spoke of his situation. The women, in response, tended to be silent or to defer to him rather than address their own needs. At the end of the last session, Philip left group feeling that his situation had not changed.

Group facilitation

The role of the facilitator is critical in pacing the group as it moves through the stages of development. Members come to the group because of the urgency of their situations. Most members have been referred by their primary care physicians due to the risk of serious illnesses related to caregiving burdens. Others identify the group as a "last resort" for support and connection. As a result, members often want to address their situations and to find solutions as quickly as possible. It is the responsibility of the facilitator to acknowledge this urgency while supporting the group and laying the foundation for the work of problem solving.

Group A is illustrative of many women-only caregiver groups that have been led by Betsey Gray, this chapter's first-named author. The group clearly illustrates the relational model of group development. In all-women groups it is important for members to get a sense of each other and to develop a level of trust and intimacy before they can challenge and confront. In Group A, when Mary initially introduced her dilemma about leaving her mother and mother-in-law in the care of others, group members responded with empathy and support and referred to similarities in their own lives. They did not challenge Mary but agreed that it must be very hard. After two meetings, one of the members gently confronted Mary about the need to take care of herself. Mary responded somewhat defensively. The group worker facilitated mutuality and interpersonal empathy by initiating a discussion about similarities in the members' caregiving situations, stating "I am wondering if others have felt this conflict." Mary was able to receive support from the other members and the challenging member was not silenced. As the group entered the mutuality and interpersonal empathy phase, group members experienced empathy with Mary's emotional pain, but did not press her to change her behavior. After several sessions had passed and the group was more cohesive, members began to challenge Mary in a manner that was supportive yet suggestive of the need for change. Mary began to use the group for problem solving and came up with a way to speak with her mother and mother-in-law about her plans for the weekend. During the course of the group, Mary did go away with her husband for a weekend and returned to say that they had had a wonderful time and that everyone had survived. Group members joined in with expressions of their support and happiness for Mary. This example clearly illustrates the worker's role in promoting mutuality and interpersonal empathy, as a prelude to challenge and change. The facilitator played a critical role in helping the group delay confrontation until it had achieved the connectedness needed to move the group forward. By validating Mary as well as the woman confronting her, the facilitator acknowledged and empathized with the similarities in their situations. Had the worker reinforced the challenge to Mary early on in the group, the members might have felt unsafe to continue, and Mary would probably have left the group. Instead, time was spent by the members getting to know one another and developing a strong relational base of support before confrontation fully occurred. As a result, Mary was able to hear the words and feel empowered to develop a plan.

In contrast, the group facilitator felt challenged by Group B, a mixed-gender caregiver support group. With hindsight, it appears that the worker's sense of inadequacy in dealing with the gender differences in this group was exacerbated by her lack of preparation. Had the group facilitator spent time examining her own gendered values and attitudes prior to the group commencing, she might have felt more confident in handling the challenges that occurred. In the case of a mixed-gender group, this involves anticipating possible reactions to both the women and the men in the group. If the facilitator is a woman, will she feel intimidated by men? Due to the historical lack of males in the caregiver groups, the facilitator of group B was accustomed to leading all-women groups through Schiller's stages of group development. Although this particular group was open to all interested caregivers, the facilitator had not fully prepared herself for the possibility of a mixed group. She neglected the step of self-examination prior to the group and was unprepared for the differences in the group related to its mixed-gender composition.

The group facilitator was surprised when the one male member confronted other members early in the group's development. Typically, in the first session of the caregivers group, the group facilitator asks members to share their caregiving situations and what they hope to achieve from the group. Following Schiller's model, the group facilitator promotes member-to-member identification at this point and directly limits confrontation so that members will have an opportunity to establish trust within the group. The group facilitator failed to accomplish this in Group B. Philip confronted some of the women during the first two meetings when they spoke of their struggles to make changes. The facilitator, in an attempt to delay confrontation and allow time for the group to establish a level of connection, as suggested in the relational model, commented on the difficulty of making change and suggested to Philip that others might find it hard to alter their situations. Philip reacted by saying, "If they want things to get better, they need to be able to fix the problem." With hindsight, the facilitator might have more actively implemented Schiller's model by drawing attention to the similarities between Philip and the other group members. It was too early in the group's development to identify the contrast implied by the facilitator's comment. The members including Philip, were feeling burdened by their caregiving tasks. The facilitator became aware that her intervention was ineffectual because the women became silent and did not challenge Philip.

Although the facilitator saw the group quickly moving to stage two of the traditional model (the power and control stage), without having established a relational base, she was unsure how to intervene. Her lack of action contributed to the very limited trust between members. Had the facilitator spent time before the group began reflecting on the impact of a male member on the group's development, she might have been able to find similarities between Philip and the other members and thus to facilitate the development of trust during these first two sessions. If she had found similarities she could have validated the experiences of the women *and* of Philip simultaneously. Validating the women without including Philip stimulated further challenging behavior. As the group progressed, the facilitator allowed the power and control issues present in the early stages of the group's development to continue unchecked. Philip often interrupted the women when they spoke and told them how they should provide care. While the facilitator acknowledged the gender differences in problem solving, her comments served to reinforce the division in the group rather than to bring it together.

Community building within the group must be facilitated *before* group workers highlight gender differences. Another way to do this is to generate the values embedded in the stories about members' caregiving situations. The following illustration from Group B may help to clarify this point. In one instance, Philip spoke of his frustration regarding his wife's illness and his isolation. He said that he wanted to enjoy his own life but felt that he couldn't. One of the women suggested he hire a nurse to relieve him so he could go out and visit friends. Philip became angry and said that he would like to but his wife "wouldn't hear of it." The woman responded with silence and the group facilitator, angered by Philip's reply, changed the subject rather than seize the opportunity to point out the similarities within the group. Instead of noting Philip's anger, the facilitator might have commented on how deeply he must care about his wife to honor her wishes. Other members in the group could identify with caring *about* as well as caring *for* their loved ones. There was a missed opportunity to facilitate mutual empathy because of the more typically male manner of presentation that derailed the group facilitator. As the group progressed, the female members focused on Philip's caregiving burdens and neglected their own. The group facilitator joined them in allowing Philip to have center stage instead of finding linkages between the other members' support of Philip and the situations they themselves were facing. Had the facilitator been aware of her own internalized sexism, she could have realized that she was deferring to Philip and neglecting her responsibility to other group members. Had adequate emphasis been placed on community building, she could have moved on to identifying the gendered issues in the group. If trust had already been developed, she could have drawn out the contrast between Philip's anger and the women's guilt. She could have noted that these differences were actually reflections of a similar bind they all felt. All members might have identified with the moral pain involved in caring for oneself while also caring about, and for, a loved one. There was also a missed opportunity to note that the lack of acceptable resources available to care receivers reflects the societal assumption that families should care for their own. At the last meeting of the group, members were very superficial in describing their progress and how the group had been helpful. Philip stated clearly that he did not feel his situation had changed. The group facilitator took this as evidence that she had not succeeded in the goal of support. Unlike Group A, members did not discuss continuing to meet as a mutual aid group. This was additional evidence to her that she had not succeeded in helping members move from support to empowerment.

We suggest that Group A was successful and Group B much less so. The members of Group A benefitted from helping Mary become more empowered to take care of herself. The members of Group B, including Philip, made no significant changes in their caregiving situations. It could be argued that the presence of the male in Group B should have immediately prompted the worker to move to a more traditional developmental model to inform her facilitation of the group. It is not clear that this approach would have yielded a more productive outcome, however, and this solution would potentially deprive mixed-gender groups of the benefits of a relational approach to group development. Rather, we propose that under most circumstances the well-planned application of Schiller's model to mixed-gender groups will enhance the likelihood of success for all members, women and men. What is required here is a paradigm shift. Rather than view the traditional model as what is considered the norm and the relational model the exception, we propose the relational model as the preferred norm in group development.

The application of feminist group work principles to practice with mixed-gender groups does entail some considerable challenges. Facilitators must find similarities between the gendered experiences of men and women within the first few sessions. A group facilitator will be more able to do this if she or he examines personal values and attitudes that may be gendered before beginning to lead a caregivers' group. Identifying the values embedded in the stories of caregivers can help point to the importance of the relationships between caregivers and care receivers. After trust is built through mutual empathy, the facilitator should consider ways to raise gender differences in a manner that validates both women and men. For example, group workers can identify differences in the ways men and women experience moral pain by contrasting the anger of men with the guilt of women. Typically, these responses emanate from similar situations. Thus both similarity and difference can be emphasized simultaneously. If challenges do arise early in women-only groups or in mixed-gender groups, workers are encouraged to facilitate delay by modeling empathy, as illustrated in Group A. Once a strong relationship base is built, gendered issues should be raised in both types of group. The identification of gendered issues is a primary method of facilitating the move from support to empowerment.

Moral dimensions of decision making

As Ann Fleck-Henderson (1998) notes, the family is a moral community. The intense feelings caregivers bring to decision making are often related to the moral dimensions of those decisions. The possibility that women may feel compelled to provide care in predetermined ways may be linked to attempts to act in a manner consistent with an ideal self grounded in "compulsory altruism" (Baines *et al.* 1991). Because shame and guilt develop when one's actions are incongruent with one's values, raising consciousness about the gendered ethical dimensions of decision making is essential if caregivers are to be confident about their decisions. As women tell their stories, group facilitators should be considering ways in which values are embedded in these stories and reflecting on how they may be gendered. Group A provides a good illustration of the way in which gendered values may be oppressive to women and may impede the recognition of their physical and emotional health needs as caregivers.

The practice examples given above illustrate the prevalence of guilt among women caregivers in contrast to the anger experienced by men. These differences may be viewed as emanating from gendered assumptions in our society about male and female roles. It is the group facilitator's responsibility to question the possibility of oppression arising from these gendered expectations. Anger arises when one is blocked from accomplishing a goal (Fiske and Taylor 1991: 434), but guilt arises when one fails to meet the expectations one holds in relation to one's ideal, or "ought," self (1991: 191–2). Given that responsibility for caring is gendered in our society, group facilitators should address the gender differences in emotional responses to caregiving that arise in the group. We should challenge the expectation that women alone will assume the responsibility for care in our society and note that the anger men experience in caregiving roles is equally associated with a lack of resources provided by society for caregiving. When a group member, such as Mary in Group A, indicates that she feels guilty about leaving her mother-in-law in the care of others for a weekend, a group facilitator may wonder whether feelings of guilt arise when we consider actions we believe are inconsistent with gendered expectations. The anger Philip expressed in group B may also be viewed as gendered, and can be likened to a woman member's guilt that similarly emanates from gendered expectations in society.

Thus, considerations of societal influence should be raised within the context of men's and women's narratives. The question to be asked is why our society does not assume shared responsibility for those who need care. As Lee (1994) indicates, group facilitators should participate in naming the oppression and moving from the personal to the political in relation to caregiving. In this way, we wonder together about public aspects of private troubles. Group members should also be encouraged to reflect upon whether the values held by others in the family, including the care receiver, are also gendered. Men in groups may assume that they are going far beyond societal expectations by becoming caregivers, while the caregiving of women may be invisible or minimized by others. Attitudes to both are stereotyped and limiting.

Conclusion

If we are to be successful in our efforts to move caregiver groups from support to empowerment by addressing societal pressures and neglect of caregiving, it is imperative that, as facilitators, we are aware of our own attitudes around gender and caregiving. We must prepare for our role as caregiver group facilitators with conscientious self-reflection concerning gendered issues. Do we buy into the norm that caregiving is predominantly a woman's job? How do our attitudes play out in our role as facilitator in caregiver groups? Do we place certain expectations on the female members but not on male members? We need to be aware of gender differences and similarities, particularly when facilitating interpersonal empathy and empowerment in caregiver groups.

We recommend that group workers actively facilitate Schiller's relational model of group development for mixed-gender groups as well as all-women groups. To fail to do so may result in both women and men leaving caregiver groups with their needs unmet. We encourage facilitators to actively bring gender issues to the surface and draw attention to the relationship between public policy and family stress in meeting the care needs of loved ones. In addition, group facilitators must address the moral pain associated with gendered values in our society that may be especially acute for women.

In summary, we recommend the following:

1   Begin with an examination of our own values and attitudes concerning gender and caregiving.
2   Build community within the group before engaging in challenge and change.
3   Together identify the values and beliefs in the story of the immediate situation.
4   Directly acknowledge the importance of relationships within the group and between the caregiver, the care receiver and the others by acknowledging that caregivers not only care *for* frail elders in their families but care very deeply *about* them.
5   Bring gender to the surface: identify the relationship between a gendered ethic of care and the distress-associated gendered responsibility for caregiving, and contrast anger and guilt.
6   Validate the moral pain involved in decision making.
7   Identify gendered values and associated inequities.
8   Identify the relationship between private troubles and public issues.
9   Raise consciousness about the dependence of society on the unpaid and low-wage labor of women.
10 Assist the group with challenging in order to move from support to empowerment.

References

Arno, P., Levine, C., and Memmott, M. (1999) "The economic value of informal care-giving," *Health Affairs*, 18, 2: 182–8.
Baines, C.T., Evans, P.M., and Neysmith, S.M. (1991) "Caring: its impact on the lives of women," in Baines, C.T., Evans, P.M., and Neysmith, S.M. (eds) *Women's Caring*, Toronto: McClelland and Stewart.

Baines, C.T., Evans, P.M., and Neysmith, S.M. (1992) "Confronting women's caring: challenges for practice and policy," *Affilia*, 7, 1: 21–44.

Briar, K.H. and Kaplan, C. (1990) *The Family Caregiving Crisis*, Silver Spring, MD: National Association of Social Workers.

Bunting, S.M. (1989) "Stress on caregivers of the elderly," *Advanced Nursing Science*, 11, 2: 63–73.

Collopy, B., Dubler, N., and Zuckerman, C. (1990) "The ethics of home care: autonomy and accommodation," *The Hastings Report*, 20, 2: 1–16.

Cox, E.O. and Parsons, R.J. (1994) *Empowerment-Oriented Social Work Practice with the Elderly*, Pacific Grove, CA: Brooks/Cole Publishing.

Fiske, S.T. and Taylor, S.E. (1991) *Social Cognition*, New York: McGraw-Hill.

Fleck-Henderson, A. (1998) "The family as moral community: a social work perspective," *Families in Society: The Journal of Contemporary Human Services*, 79, 3: 233–40.

Garland, J., Jones, H., and Kolodney, R. (1965) "A model for stages of development in social work groups," in Bernstein, S. (ed.) *Exploration in Group Work: Essays in Theory and Practice*, Boston, MA: Boston University School of Social Work.

Gilligan, C. (1983) *In a Different Voice*, Cambridge, MA: Harvard University Press.

Lee, J.A. (1994) *The Empowerment Approach to Social Work Practice*, New York: Columbia University Press.

Miller, J.B. (1977) *Toward a New Psychology of Women*, Boston, MA: Beacon Press.

Office of Management and Budget Watch (1990) "*Long Term Care Policy: Where Are We Going?*", Boston: Gerontology Institute, University of Massachusetts.

Scheyett, A. (1990) "The oppression of caring: women caregivers of relatives with mental illness," *Affilia*, 5, 1: 32–48.

Schiller, L.Y. (1997) "Rethinking stages of development in women's groups: implications for practice", *Social Work With Groups*, 20, 3: 3–19.

Siegel, J.S. (1993) *A Generation of Change: Profile of America's Older Population*, New York: Russell Sage Foundation.

Toseland, R.W. (1995) *Group Work with the Elderly and Family Caregivers*, New York: Springer.

Toseland, R.W. and Rivas, R.F. (2001) *An Introduction to Group Work Practice*, Boston, MA: Allyn & Bacon.

Ungerson, C. (1983) "Why do women care?" in Finch, J. and Groves, D. (eds) *A Labour of Love*, London: Routledge & Kegan Paul.

Chapter 13

Challenges and issues facing older women

Potential role for empowerment-oriented groups

Alberta Dooley and Enid Opal Cox

This chapter focuses on the context and process of empowerment-oriented group work with elderly women. The significance of gender as it impacts group work with older women is explored. The insights offered by critical gerontology and feminist practice are outlined and future challenges to empowerment-oriented group practice suggested. The intervention examples are drawn from experience with pilot empowerment projects conducted through the University of Denver's Institute of Gerontology and all statistics are US-specific.

The politics of gender

The recognition that ageism is a gendered process is critical in understanding the current political discourse on an ageing population (Arber and Ginn 1991). To ignore or to fail to acknowledge the gender differences in the ageing process is to risk implementing ineffectual intervention strategies and, at the very least, to perpetuate the status quo. An analysis of gender is especially relevant in empowerment-oriented practice with older women that emphasizes ageing as a women's issue. By virtue of their gender and socially prescribed gender roles and expectations, women in late life often lack the resources they need. The focus brought by feminists on the relationship of caregiving throughout the life span, disadvantaged labor market participation, and inequality in retirement opportunities, is an acknowledgment of how gender bias contributes to late life differences between women and men.

Older women in general provide a powerful illustration of great strength, incredible resilience, and social contribution. Elderly women have survived the consequences of sexism and, modified by personal fate or fortune, of classism, racism, and homophobia. Ageism imposes another layer of discrimination to women's efforts to secure quality of life for themselves and others. As Arber and Ginn (1991: 50) argue, "the debate over the significance of an ageing population has been flawed by the neglect of gender differences."

Feminist gerontologists have contrasted the conceptualization of caregiver stress as a woman's private responsibility with the way in which gendered structural arrangements of work and caregiving create women's dependence and low-income status (Hooyman 1999). Empowerment-oriented groups are often challenged to address this issue from the standpoint of both caregivers and care receivers. Women's issues with late life caregiving also raise questions of the impact of current policy and program focus on "productive ageing", both in how that is defined and in the implications of this theme for policy and the creation of the future moral economy of ageing.

Finally, social roles of older women that are created within the current political and economic structure must be critically analyzed as they apply to late life. Ideas about beauty, definitions of family (primary support networks), the role of men as caregivers, accepting care when needed, and employment arenas for older women need to be addressed. In sum, feminist thought and analysis has much to add to critical gerontology as it grows with the assistance of scholars and of older women.

Theoretical frameworks

The critical gerontology framework described by Townsend (1986), Phillipson (1991), Ovrebo and Minkler (1993), Estes (1999), and many other scholars provides an insightful and dynamic guide for on-going analysis of issues facing elderly women. These insights have been informed by group interventions with older women, and have helped workers and their clients as they have struggled together to understand various aspects of late life challenges. Critical gerontology includes a political economy and a moral economy perspective that increasingly recognize the experience of ageing as perceived by the elders themselves. The inclusion of feminist and cultural/ethnic perspectives is integral to both political and moral economy considerations for critical gerontologists. The questions raised are often akin to those that emerge from consciousness-raising activity in groups of older women. Critical gerontology when applied to empowerment-oriented group work provides a knowledge base for understanding "how lifelong differences in resources will affect health and well-being and the ways in which coping strategies will vary greatly by gender, race, ethnicity, and so forth" (Minkler 2000: 451).

Empowerment-oriented and feminist group work practice models

Emerging empowerment-oriented and feminist models of group work practice share many values and strategies. One important common phenomenon is the emergence of a variety of approaches which present themselves as either feminist or empowerment-oriented while being rooted in very different philosophies and political perspectives. The models discussed here as related to the needs of older women are those rooted in the critical perspective of ageing and feminist perspectives outlined above. Specifically, they are rooted in the recognition of the impact of class, ethnicity, racism, disability, ageism and participation in same-sex unions on late life status and challenges (Bricker-Jenkins 2000). The key area of difference among these models is the greater attention to patriarchy and a more exclusive focus on women's issues. Common components of these models are suggested below.

Lee's eight principles of empowerment (1994) apply to many feminist practice models as well as serving to ground workers in the politics of gender. Lee emphasizes the importance of workers challenging all oppression, maintaining holistic vision and a focus on the person as victor not victim, and of maintaining a social change focus. Lee further suggests that people in similar circumstances or those who share "common ground" will benefit from working together to attain power. This is particularly relevant to group work with older women. Group workers need to be acutely aware of the political history of the role that gender has played in the lives of older women. This knowledge is essential to assist older women in developing trust, a sense of their own power, and a change focus.

Bricker-Jenkins (2000), while embracing the need for a change focus, raises concerns from a feminist perspective that also guides practice. She notes the need to distinguish between what is political practice, pertaining to distributions of power, and what is transformational practice, pertaining to changes in the nature of power as well as its distributions. These principles include the strengths-based essence of both empowerment-oriented and feminist practice models, and they set an excellent framework for group work practice interventions.

Worker role in empowerment-oriented practice with elderly women

Group interventions have long been the preferred method of intervention for empowerment-oriented social workers (Mullender and Ward 1991; Breton 1994; Cox and Parsons 1994; Lee 1994; Gutiérrez et al. 1998; Cohen and Mullender 1999). Essential group processes for empowerment, according to Cox and Parsons (1994), include:

- identifying and sharing common problems, needs, and goals;
- exploiting the group's collective intelligence through sharing of facts, experiential knowledge, and ways of coping;
- providing mutual support;
- participating in consciousness-raising experiences regarding the personal and political dimensions of the issues being considered;
- providing on-going personal support;
- accomplishing as a group goals that cannot be accomplished by individuals alone;
- providing a network for collective political action; and
- engaging in social action activities.

Empowerment and feminist interventions often share:

- an emphasis on a holistic approach to problem or issue analysis, including personal and political aspects, including an emphasis on strengths;
- a positive focus on diversity;
- the use of consciousness-raising as a primary intervention strategy;
- an emphasis on collectivity and social action as key to changing life circumstances that are presented by clients as problematic; and
- egalitarian worker–client relationships (see Cox 1989; Gutiérrez 1990; Breton 1994; Lee 1994; Gutiérrez et al. 1998; Bricker-Jenkins 2000; Cox and Parsons 2000).

Empowerment-oriented groups with older women described in the literature include these characteristics. Groups have provided a place where older women have the opportunity to explore both their real political circumstances and attitudes related to those circumstances, including their own (Cox 1989; McNicoll and Christensen 1993; Mok and Mui 1996; McInnis-Dittrich 1997; Cox 2002). Groups also provide the site for educational activity, self-help activity, and social action often occuring simultaneously (Cox 1989). As issues are taken on by the group, both the personal and political aspects are addressed (Cohen and Mullender 2000). Strengths-based assessment and practice are facilitated by groups as individual members share their histories, coping strategies, and skills. Sharing of individual resources leads to a positive valuing of diversity, as individuals from different backgrounds identify common issues, needs, and struggles, learn from each other, and collectively take action (engaging in self-help, social support, or social action, activities together). The next section of this chapter describes brief excerpts of group work with older women in two arenas of interest: care receiving challenges and late life employment issues. In general, the observations offered are based on work over the past fifteen years sponsored by the University of Denver's Institute of Gerontology (IOG).

Group work and care receiving

Context

There are few empowerment-oriented interventions that target elderly persons who have lost physical and mental capacity to the point of requiring personal care in order to accomplish the activities of daily living. Often the focus is on caregiver needs or on ways to provide specific assistance to elders. A few social workers have developed empowerment-oriented interventions targeting elders who require caregivers (Cox and Parsons 1994; McInnis-Dittrich 1997). Efforts in this area are increasing, however, as the medical and related professions have become more aware of the critical role of self-care in health outcomes (Spitzer et al. 1996; Stoller 1998). Themes that are often raised with respect to care receiving, from the perspective of elderly persons receiving care (gained from qualitative studies and from group intervention experience), include:

- concerns regarding increasing dependence;
- need for knowledge about health and social resources;
- interest in knowledge and skills related to self-care (including strategies for maintaining mental health);
- issues related to communication with personal and political caregivers;
- issues related to survival resources (income, housing, medical care, and medicine, etc.);
- ways of assisting caregivers; and
- issues related to meaning in life and death (Cox in press).

Another dimension of the critical gerontology perspective of which group workers need to be aware encompasses insights generated through exploration of the "ageing enterprise". These include the "social creation of dependency of older persons" and the "bio-medicalization of ageing" (Estes 1999: 136). The ageing enterprise is defined by Carol Estes (1999: 136) as "programs, organizations, bureaucracies, interest groups, trade associations, providers, industries, and professionals that serve the aged in one capacity or another." One phenomenon related to analysis of the ageing enterprise that provides important understandings for both older women and group workers is the social creation of dependence. Estes identifies several forces that have promoted dependence:

> social policies and practice that permit age discrimination and, until recently, mandatory retirement, lower incomes of retired persons that decline with age, high and growing out-of-pocket health care costs that are not offset by Medicare or Social Security, the treatment of functional disability and chronic disease with acute medical care rather than rehabilitative and personal support, the discrimination and exclusion of elders from multiple arenas of social life precipitated by loss of social contacts through retirement, widowhood, and the death of friends, low self-esteem and lack of confidence resulting from the stigmatized status of older persons and the asymmetrical power relations between older persons and the professional caregivers who provide them services
>
> (1999: 137)

Analysis by group workers from this critical gerontology perspective provides valuable insights to empowerment-oriented practitioners as they engage in collaborative analysis and action with their older women clients. The critical perspectives outlined above provide group workers with the tools needed for effective work with older women. As the following excerpts illustrate, the politics of both ageing and gender must be understood and addressed to effectively join with and facilitate the quandaries facing older women.

Excerpts

The following excerpts are focused primarily on the issue of rethinking dependence in late life. A group of elderly women who required care was developed near three low-income apartment houses in downtown Denver. Meetings were held at a church that was located directly across the street from these apartment facilities and was disability accessible. Twelve elderly women of mixed ethnicity were recruited through flyers posted in the buildings and through direct visits by the group worker. The first concern raised by the group was related to building safety. Members were concerned about locks and lighting (lighting concerns were especially related to the safety of caregivers). One member had been involved in a residents' advisory committee for a public housing facility when she was younger. She shared some of her landlord-negotiating experiences with the group and assumed some group leadership. Over the first few weeks the group planned and implemented a number of actions related to safety issues, resulting in better lighting and new safety locks in all three buildings, a better call system in two buildings, and several self-help systems. The self-help systems involved organizing a number of residents in each building who would walk visitors to their cars after dark and others who undertook group shopping. During weekly meetings focused on safety, however, other issues emerged, such as: worries about causing problems for their caregivers; transportation concerns; difficulties related to health care, and other subjects. As concern for safety lessened, the group decided to spend some time on health care issues. Interestingly, the first meeting scheduled to address such issues led to a discussion about members' struggles with increasing dependence.

This topic was predominant for the next several meetings. Key themes and the related actions were as follows: in the initial discussion many revealed their surprise at this turn of events – "I never thought about having a stroke"; "I was always in good health until I turned 90, but who thought I would be 90?"; "I planned to work until I dropped dead, but now I can't even walk to the store" – and their extreme dislike of being more dependent – "I always prayed that my children would not have to take care of me"; "I hoped I would be dead before I needed care. I hate taking help from anyone; I was always the one who gave help"; "I am angry all the time"; "I try to do all I can, but I feel like I am a burden: I don't like to take help from others but I have to." Rationales for accepting assistance included: "I don't like it; it's hard but, she [her daughter] wants to help me"; "I didn't like it at first – but I know I need it, so it's OK"; "I've helped a lot of people"; "I took care of my mother. I think older women deserve respect and assistance from their children." And there were declarations of immediate reciprocity – "I try to do all I can to help them [her caregivers], with love and money"; "I babysit and do any ironing and housework I can when I am at her [granddaughter's] house." The second meeting focused on women and caregiving. Participants began to review lifelong contributions to caregiving, civic contributions (such as work for churches, schools and other community work) and to paid employment – "It seems I have

been busy every day of my life, whether other people saw me as working or not";
"We should not be so poor from all this work. I think we deserve better income";
"We shouldn't have to beg for health care and medicine"; "If we had transportation,
she [her niece] wouldn't have to come so often."

These conversations led to an analysis of ideas about independence/dependence
and finally back to health care and social service programs, resulting in further
group actions (for example, writing to the director of an unresponsive seniors'
health care facility, accompanying each other to health care appointments, etc.).

Group work and older women workers

Context

Older workers find themselves facing age discrimination, often from their forties
onward. Older women represent approximately 70 percent of older persons living
in poverty in the USA while almost half of older African American women
experience poverty. Primary income sources (often fixed) include social security,
supplemental security income, income from assets, pensions, and employment.
Income from all these sources is less available to women (Hooyman and Kiyak
1999). Current estimates suggest that women's wages are about 70 percent of
men's. Older women are finding that the labor market remains hostile to their
efforts to secure well-paying jobs. While larger proportions of women at all ages
below 65 in the USA are in the paid workforce, life/work patterns continue to reflect
interrupted employment, low-paying positions and difficult work that does not
challenge the employee or provide learning opportunities that lead to advancement
(Hatch 1990). Gender inequality is perhaps most evident in the differences in
pension wealth that exist between men and women. Some studies report differen-
tials as high as 76 percent greater wealth in favor of men (Johnson et al. 1999).

Work and training programs have been available sporadically, but few comprehensive interventions that address all aspects of work and women's lives are
available. The term "empowerment" is often used in discussing work-related
programming, but the meaning is often limited to empowerment through employment. Themes emerging from empowerment-oriented groups with older women
include: age discrimination; fear of technology; low wages; vulnerability in office
situations; limitations on jobs considered open to women; difficulties with training;
home responsibilities; and transportation resources (Dooley 1996).

The excerpts from group discussions that follow come from ten older (55–79
years) women of different ethnic backgrounds who were participating in a seniors'
community employment program targeting low-income older people. The
program provided limited training (interview skills, basic office relationship
skills) and on-the-job training. It is important to note that several of the members
were placed in human service agencies. This training was limited to one year
(occasionally extended to two) and paid the minimum wage for a twenty-hour
working week.

Excerpts

The group met for one year under a pilot empowerment grant. The first three sessions were spent discussing the program, including its pros and cons. Negatives included: low wages; the one-year cut off (participants were expected to find permanent employment within the year); problems with staff who were perceived as disrespectful; the need to slow down the training pace (especially for those who received on-the-job technology training); insecure job futures (many had been in search of employment for years prior to finding this program). The positives far outweighed the negatives. They included an increased sense of personal worth: "You feel valuable, worth a damn"; "I like the power in working, being employed"; "I have Lupus, and without this I would not get up in the morning. I [now] have something important to do." Other positive aspects were an enhanced status in the family – "My kids learn from me: one was having trouble with his supervisor, and I was able to advise him on his relationship with his boss"; "My grandkids look up to me now: one said he told everyone in school that his grandmother was employed in a good job" – and meaningful work – "I can't believe that I get paid to help people; that's what I like to do"; "I have been working in a hospital, [and] now older people are asking for advice from me. I guess they feel I understand."

In later meetings, the themes changed to ways to improve the program, how to develop permanent jobs, barriers to older women, and ways to maintain a permanent support group. Four members joined the local Older Women's League, and the group began to participate in social action strategies.

These brief illustrations demonstrate the potential for engaging elderly women in empowerment processes through group interventions. Knowledge of how gender has affected the circumstances of the older women in the groups is a critical component for effective empowerment group work practice. Awakening gender consciousness in members of the group decreases self-blame, increases self-esteem, and contributes to identification with the group (Rinehart 1992). Many empowerment groups, including those described above, continue after formal program efforts cease.

Worker role

Empowerment-oriented workers in these and other groups piloted at the IOG were responsible for recruiting the groups. Workers explained that empowerment-oriented groups focus on issues of concern to potential participants and include education, mutual support, and social action. The strengths-based focus was also explored. Worker tasks included finding locations for at least the initial meetings and encouraging a revolving meeting leadership where possible. They participated with other groups in finding resources (such as speakers, expert opinion, knowledge about service delivery systems and educational materials, etc.) and shared knowledge based on their particular expertise and experience, as do all group members.

Perhaps the most critical role of the worker relates to the consciousness-raising process. Workers encourage the group members to identify common issues and experiences (especially as older women), as well as unique experiences, and to explore both personal and political aspects of issues raised. Workers will share ideas and questions that have been generated by older women in other projects. Members are asked for their permission to allow their insights, strategies, and other knowledge that is generation-related to be shared with other groups, as more empowerment-oriented group projects are developed (Cox 2002). Overall, workers strive to develop egalitarian relationships with group members and to work toward group-generated goals.

Challenges and future strategies for groups with older women

The development and use of group work strategies with older women face strong resistance at the policy and service delivery design levels, as suggested by the perspectives of critical gerontology outlined above. The medicalization of ageing, deep cuts in social service programs, age discrimination, and other factors result in social service delivery systems that are under-funded and inappropriately designed. Most intervention sites focus on direct service, and the worker role is often defined as "case management." While case management can cover a variety of services, these are seldom empowerment-oriented and groups are rare. Existing groups are often limited to specific content education and or social/emotional support. Empowerment-oriented social workers are challenged to change policy and develop funding for programs that engage older women in empowerment groups. A wide variety of sites, including assisted living facilities, nursing homes, senior rental facilities, neighborhoods with congregated senior populations, recreation centers, and senior clinics, provide appropriate settings for group interventions.

Program-level challenges include the need to increase training in empowerment strategies in schools of social work and in agencies, with special attention to critical gerontology and feminist thought. Increased attention and resources are also needed to describe and evaluate these interventions in a form that facilitates replication. Empowerment-oriented group work, informed by the theoretical framework and perspectives discussed above, has great potential for confronting and improving the conditions facing older women and revitalizing their capacity to be proactive participants in determining the quality of their lives.

References

Arber, S. and Ginn, J. (1991) *Gender and Later Life*, Newbury Park, CA: Sage.
Breton, M. (1994) "On the meaning of empowerment and empowerment-oriented practice," *Social Work With Groups*, 17, 3: 23–37.
Bricker-Jenkins, M. (2000) "Feminist social work practice: womanly warrior or damsel in

distress?" in Allen-Meares, P. and Garvin, C. (eds) *Handbook of Social Work Direct Practice*, Thousand Oaks, CA: Sage.

Cohen, M. and Mullender, A. (2000) "The personal in the political: exploring the group work continuum from individual to social change goals", *Social Work With Groups*, 22, 1: 13–31.

Cox, E.O. (1989) "Empowerment of the low income elderly through group work," *Social Work With Groups*, 39, 3: 262–8.

—— (2002) "Empowerment-oriented practice applied to long term care," *Journal of Social Work in Long Term Care*, 1, 2: 27–46.

Cox, E.O. and Parsons, R.J. (1994) *Empowerment-Oriented Social Work Practice with the Elderly*, Pacific Grove, CA: Brooks/Cole.

Cox, E.O. and Parsons, R. (2000) "Empowerment-practice: from practice value to practice model", in Allen-Meares, P. and Garvin, C. (eds) *The Handbook of Social Work Direct Practice*, Thousand Oaks, CA: Sage.

Dooley, A. (1996) "Senior community service employment programs," unpublished doctoral dissertation, University of Denver, Denver, CO.

Estes, C. (1999) "Critical gerontology and the new political economy of aging," in Minkler, M. and Estes, C. (eds) *Critical Gerontology: Perspectives and Political and Moral Economy*, Amityville, New York: Baywood.

Gutiérrez, L. (1990) "Working with women of color: an empowerment perspective", *Social Work*, 35, 2: 149–53.

Gutiérrez, L., Parsons, R., and Cox, E. (1998) *Empowerment in Social Work Practice: A Source Book*, Pacific Grove, CA: Brooks/Cole.

Hatch, L. (1990) "Gender and work at midlife and beyond," *Generations*, 14, 3: 48–52.

Hooyman, N. (1999) "Book review," *Gerontologist*, 39, 1: 115–18.

Hooyman, N. and Kiyak, H. (1999) *Social Gerontology: A Multidisciplinary Perspective*, Boston, MA: Allyn & Bacon.

Johnson, R., Sambamoorthi, U. and Crystal, S. (1999) "Gender differences in pension wealth: estimates using provider data," *Gerontologist*, 39, 3: 320–33.

Lee, J.A.B. (1994) *The Empowerment Approach to Social Work Practice*, New York: Columbia University Press.

McInnis-Dittrich, K. (1997) "An empowerment-oriented mental health intervention with elderly Appalachian women: the women's club," *Journal of Women and Aging* 9, 1–2: 91–105.

McNicoll, P. and Christensen, C. (1993) "Making changes and making sense: social work groups with Vietnamese older people," Paper presented at the 15th Symposium of the Association for the Advancement of Social Work with Groups, New York City.

Minkler, M. (2000) "New challenges for gerontology", in Markson, E.M. and Hollis-Sawyer, L. (eds) *Intersections of Aging: Readings in Social Gerontology*, Los Angeles, CA: Roxbury.

Mok, B. and Mui, A. (1996) "Empowerment in residential care for the elders: the case of an aged home in Hong Kong," *Journal of Gerontological Social Work*, 27, 1–2: 23–35.

Mullender, A. and Ward, D. (1991) *Self-Directed Groupwork: Users Take Action for Empowerment*, London: Whiting & Birch.

Ovrebo, Z.B. and Minkler, M. (1993) "The lives of older women: perspectives from political economy and the humanities," in Cole, T., Achenbaum, A., Jakobi, P., and Kastenbaum, R. (eds) *Voices and Visions of Aging: Towards a Critical Gerontology*, New York: Springer Publishing Company.

Phillipson, C. (1991) "The social construction of old age: perspectives from political economy", *Reviews in Clinical Gerontology*, 19, 2: 27–36.

Rinehart, S. (1992) *Gender Consciousness and Politics*, London: Routledge.

Spitzer, A., Bar-Tal, Y. and Ziv, L. (1996) "The moderating effect of age on self-care," *Western Journal of Nursing Research*, 18, 2: 136–48.

Stoller, E. (1998) "Dynamics and processes of self-care in old age," in Ory, M. and DeFriese, G. (eds) *Self-Care in Later Life: Research, Program, and Policy Issues*, New York: Springer.

Townsend, P. (1986) "Ageism and social policy", in Phillipson, C. and Walker, A. (eds) *Ageing and Social Policy: A Critical Assessment*, Aldershot: Gower.

Chapter 14

Grouping together for equality in physical health

Eileen McLeod

Introduction

Networks of feminist groups focusing on health issues, as part of a widespread grassroots women's movement, have disappeared in the UK. However, significant groupwork initiatives addressing gendered health issues continue to develop in a more disparate form (McLeod and Bywaters 2000). Important in their own right, these initiatives also contribute to propelling groupwork practice forward. This chapter examines present trends as exemplified in a recent initiative: the first facilitated self-help support group in the UK specifically for older women with secondary breast cancer (SBC) where cure is no longer possible (Baum *et al.* 1995). Drawing on interviews with group members about their group experience, major lessons from this development include:

- evidence of how sexism interacting with further dimensions to social inequality is reflected in daunting problems associated with ill-health, including social isolation and subordinating contact with health care professionals;
- confirmation that groupwork can be a source of empowerment for securing a more equal chance of well-being in ill-health;
- recognition that groupwork needs to address how it can also be a site of social inequality to the detriment of members' well-being.

Antecedents

A gendered map of health

Current UK groupwork addressing gender and physical health has antecedents in feminist groups organizing on health in the 1970s as an integral part of second-wave feminism (Doyal 1995). They put gender and health on the map of public affairs in three main ways. First, they uncovered how patriarchal social relations undermined women's health and their well-being in ill-health (Collins *et al.* 1978). Second, women challenged unequal power relations permeating health care, characterized by a male-dominated medical profession (Greenwood and Young

1976). Third, women created valuable new resources for self-help health care (MacKeith 1978).

Further development: process

Group process in early and subsequent groups tackling gendered health issues cannot be characterized as either/or consciousness-raising, campaigning, self-help, or support giving. Even where groups identified themselves as taking one of these forms, different elements of group process tended to be interwoven (Collins *et al.* 1978). This characteristic fusion of different forms of group process continues, as in Positively Women's work on HIV AIDS which combines peer support, drop-in centre facilities and pressure-group activities (Positively Women 1994).

A close reading of earlier accounts also reveals that women professionals contributed to supporting and facilitating groups, even if the primary impetus came from a self-help movement. Evidence of such alliances continues. Now, typically, paid women community health workers, committed to women securing greater equity in health, aim to assist women residents organizing on a locality basis. But, as was the case then (see Finch 1982), the question persists as to whether professional and class differences can lead to control over a group's working agenda against the interests of women members (Bywaters and McLeod 1996).

Further development: issues

Groups may continue to focus primarily on physical health issues. However, recognizing that these are inextricably bound up with psychological well-being remains a hallmark of a feminist approach. Through sharing their experiences, women have, for example, helped to pinpoint insidious forms of social exclusion that undermine their psychological well-being when going through the menopause (Granville 2000), and the need for the process of stillbirth to be open to grieving (Littlewood 1992).

The major challenge to the agenda of groupwork addressing gendered health issues has come from collective action against other oppressions. This has brought growing recognition that tackling inequality means recognizing the extent to which sexism is permeated by other dimensions to social disadvantage (Saulnier 2000). In the UK, activists developing older people's self-help health care, for example, have focused on the impact of ageism on women's health (Bernard 2000). Groupwork promoting health care access among women from minority ethnic groups has highlighted the need to confront institutionalized racism as well as gendered caring responsibilities (Weaver 1996). Self-help/support groups representing populations experiencing specific forms of ill-health have also proliferated, to equalize service user–professional power relations (Gott *et al.* 2000). Meanwhile, tackling the impact of different dimensions of social disadvantage on health has become a central issue in academic discourse and health policy. This has uncovered the fundamental association between poverty and reduced life-expectancy, higher chances of serious illness, and inferior treatment in ill-health (Graham 2000).

Older women and secondary breast cancer

Group origins

The specific initiative featured here is a microcosm of these intertwined tendencies in current groupwork on gender and health. The hospice social workers who set up the group identified it as a 'union of women'. Nevertheless, although the existing developments they drew on aimed to promote women's well-being, they also challenged disablist and ageist social exclusion:

* C4Ward – an alliance of women with secondary breast cancer (SBC), volunteers and professionals – pioneered the UK development of facilitated self-help support groups for women with SBC. C4Ward originated in the determination of Alison McCartney to experience group support with women in the same situation. She had found that the needs of terminally ill women such as herself could not be met in a group focusing principally on recovery (McCartney 1995). Together with a breast care nurse counsellor, McCartney set up the original group in the C4Ward network (Lockett 1996). Since 1997, C4Ward has been under the management of Breast Cancer Care – a national voluntary organization offering information and support to those affected by breast cancer.
* Age Concern's anti-ageist campaign across the late 1990s, to extend routine invitation to breast cancer screening in the UK to women aged over 65, brought to public attention that the majority of deaths from breast cancer occur in this age group (Age Concern England 1996). A feasibility survey for the group highlighted here showed that its target population – women aged over 60 with SBC – represented 20 per cent of the hospice's service users.

Group identity

This account draws on a study of group members and facilitators across the initial six months of the C4Ward group in 1998 (for a detailed report see McLeod 2000). Planned as open-ended, the group has met fortnightly since then and is still running. It is open to any woman over 60 with SBC, using any of the hospice's services, and is facilitated by a hospice social worker and a volunteer. In a pattern common to groups in cancer care (Hitch *et al.* 1994), it aims to combine self-help and support, with members retaining a high degree of direction over group aims and activities but with professional input in establishing the group and facilitating discussion.

At the time of the interviews, the eight group members were aged between 63 and 84. The length of time since their diagnosis of SBC varied between one and three years. With the exception of one woman, who lived alone, members lived either with their husband or an adult child. As is characteristic of the majority of pensioners living in relative poverty, who are women (Falkingham 1998), their current income level was very low, averaging £75–£95 per week. Most lived in a household without a car. All described themselves as white, English.

Daunting demands of ill-health and inequality

All group members were coping with daunting physical, emotional and social demands associated with their illness. However, their experience also reflected the imprint of gendered, ageist/disablist social relations and relative poverty on ill-health.

Physical symptoms

Everyone in the group was grappling with the variety of physical symptoms associated with SBC (Baum *et al.* 1995). The pain could be intense, and, prior to hospice care, the women's experience also testified to the absence of comprehensive pain relief in an overstretched National Health Service (Addington Hall and McCarthy 1993).

> One day I just could not get out of bed, I screamed and I cried. My husband couldn't get me out, I couldn't get out . . . and I said 'Just leave me . . . get one of my painkillers.' . . . It took about an hour after that before the pain had gone sufficiently to allow me to get out of bed.
>
> (Beryl)

Women also identified a profound degree of physical impairment arising from fatigue and debility. None of them used a wheelchair all the time but most could walk only short distances unaided and in some cases could not climb stairs. Persistent and acute breathlessness, which women found very worrying and restrictive, featured prominently. Mary's experience also illustrates how limited income could exacerbate the problem of breathlessness, and ageist discrimination delay pain relief. As Mary commented: 'When you're breathless like I am, how am I going to get to the doctor's? It's two buses up there because of the hills.' And, concerning the practice nurse's initial response to her experience of bony metastases (secondary tumours), Mary related a conversation in which she said to the nurse, '"Oh my bones ache." She says "Well, how old are your bones, Mary?" I said, "Eighty-four." She says, "Well, what are you saying? Mine are 47 years old and mine ache as well." So that was putting it in its place.'

Emotional demands

Women felt a wide range of negative emotional reactions to their condition, including revulsion, depression, fear and a sense of loss. Lily, on her response to her mastectomy scar, said: 'I just couldn't look at it and couldn't even touch it . . . I couldn't.' Hilary insisted the interview went ahead but was tearful throughout, describing it as 'how she was'. Even where women had close family, they were isolated because they felt other people couldn't understand what they were going through without sharing their experience. Janet commented: 'You can't talk to your family about things you can talk about to other people who have gone through the same situation.'

Besides managing the emotional demands of their own ill-health, women retained the worry of gendered responsibilities as carers. Croft (1996) has demonstrated that women with life-threatening illnesses continue in the role of carer. This was certainly evident here: for example, Janet remained her brother's main carer, while Lily was preoccupied with her adult son's psychological problems.

Need for additional social resources

While coping with intense physical and emotional demands, women also needed additional social and material resources. No one complained, but their accounts reflected the under-funded nature of the public services they relied on for vital homecare. Hospital social workers had put in some key provisions but, in each case where a woman had profound physical impairment, others were lacking. Frances, for example, had a walking stick and a commode but lacked ramps and a stair-lift. Women's low income precluded private social care as an alternative.

Friends were seen as crucial, helping to make life worth living through companionship. Sadly, however, women's accounts revealed that they tended to have limited access to close friends, identified as providing a major source of emotional support to women (O'Connor 1992). Ageist/disablist social norms and low income combined to restrict supportive social contact.

> I'd like someone I could go out with a bit . . . what with getting older like me, [friends] just don't come out a lot. (Lily)

> I don't really see anybody much . . . two friends popped in last Wednesday but it might be weeks, months, before I see them again, because they're both elderly: 84, 85. They both come on buses. (Mary)

Mutual support: more equal chances of well-being in ill-health

Feedback from the group suggests that, primarily through the growth of reciprocal support and solidarity underwritten by facilitators' input, a facilitated self-help support group can contribute to more equal chances of well-being in ill-health. This group was not a campaigning group nor, as documented for some facilitated self-help support groups focusing on health issues, did it act as a springboard for campaigning (Gott et al. 2000). Nevertheless, the mutual aid and enhanced resources it offered redressed social disadvantage in incremental ways. As Cohen and Mullender (1999) have argued, such achievements should merit recognition as being on the continuum of social change.

Mutual support: each other's key worker

Women endorsed a theme central to feminist groupwork, but also to self-help/support groups in palliative care (Monroe 1997) and the service users' movement (Croft and Beresford 1997). They most valued group participation for providing mutual support grounded in what they defined as shared first-hand experience. They identified each other as 'key workers' and the main characteristics of such support as:

- being met with a deeper level of understanding;
- enabling each other to express more freely what they were going through; and
- gaining a sense of solidarity from realizing other people were in a similar situation.

Mutual support helped in dealing with physical symptoms, emotional demands and the need for additional social resources, associated with SBC but permeated by social inequalities.

Dealing with physical symptoms

In keeping with the feminist groupwork tradition, and with self-help health-care groups more generally (Manor 1999), the group functioned as a comprehensive 'information exchange'.

> We've gone through the whole process . . . the chemotherapy and how that's affected people, the radiotherapy . . . how to manage some of the discomforts and problems that arise after treatment has ceased. I mean, there's been a lot of fluid in their arms (lymphoedema) and they've discussed how they coped with that.
>
> (Sue, facilitator)

Group solidarity helped even up doctor–patient power imbalances (National Cancer Alliance 1996) as facilitators and group members encouraged some women to request more adequate pain relief when reluctant to 'trouble the doctor'. Paradoxically, group members also described gaining a sense of solidarity from finding that ageist treatment in the course of health care was a common experience (Age Concern England 1999).

The facilitators tried to remove disablist barriers to participation. They were conscious that more remained to be done: for example, hearing amplification was unavailable. Group members testified to the essential nature of measures that were in place. Several commented that free transport to and from the group was crucial to participating. All found the meeting room accessible. The timing, length and frequency of meetings – mid morning, for ninety minutes with refreshments served, fortnightly – were manageable.

Support for emotional demands

Both group members and facilitators described how reciprocal support, grounded in shared experience of SBC, helped lift women's spirits. Olive observed: 'Meeting other women who've been in the same position and to hear how they're coping, it helps you a lot.' The group also provided the chance to discuss searing dilemmas in close relationships, such as one group member's sadness at having to sleep separately from her partner of forty years because of the intense pain of any physical contact.

A recurrent theme in groupwork in palliative care is the risk of intensifying emotional distress because of the focus on dying (Firth 2000). This group's experience confirms that such intensification does not necessarily happen. Women described how participating in the group had actually helped in addressing fears of death. Death being close was not a constant theme in discussion. It tended to be talked about when women were particularly aware of it as an issue, for example at follow-up appointments or when acutely depressed. But – as noted in similar groups (see e.g. Burch 1997) – women described gaining some reassurance from a stronger sense of solidarity in facing death in the foreseeable future. 'You do wonder if you are the only one who has horrible feelings and depressions. It's good to be able to discuss things with people in similar positions.'

The group did not challenge gendered expectations of caring responsibilities. However, women identified other members' appreciation of the heavy nature of such demands, from their own experience, as a great morale booster. The group was also a mine of information and advice. For example, one group member took up the suggestion of counselling for her son with severe psychological problems, which proved very helpful.

Group members were divided about advantages to a group solely for older women, one pointing out that from the 80-year-old's vantage point, 60 was 'younger'. But several identified closer rapport and a sense of pride, together with some protection from ageism, as advantageous. The group was welcomed as an opportunity for socializing. As Winnie remarked: 'Oh, yes, we're not always downhearted – we do have a laugh.'

Help with additional resources

In common with other facilitated self-help support groups for people with life-threatening illnesses (McLeod 1998), this group boosted low income and shortcomings in state care services. This was particularly important, given the gendered nature of relative poverty in old age to which group members were prey (see also Chapter 13, this volume, by Dooley and Cox). Group members encouraged each other to claim social security benefits. Facilitators built in regular slots on benefit entitlements and accessed care. Frances observed: 'I found it ever so beneficial. . . . I couldn't get a chiropodist but they managed to arrange one. They also got an OT [occupational therapist] to organize ramps between rooms.' Poignantly, some group members could not afford a holiday and facilitators tried to obtain funds for that purpose: 'At least three members of the group haven't had a holiday since goodness knows when, but weren't in a position income-wise to go. . . . Given everything they are going through, they could do with a break' (Jenny).

These accounts of group interaction illustrate how membership of a facilitated self-help support group may help to combat the negative impact of sexism in interaction with other dimensions of inequality in the course of illness. They add to the case for considering such groups as a potent resource for greater equity in health.

A site of social inequality

Despite these positive attributes, feedback also shows how such groups are not immune to discriminatory tendencies in wider social relations. This needs to be addressed in the interests of the health of current and potential members.

Racism

As in palliative care services more generally (Oliviere *et al.* 1998), racist barriers to access existed. The proportion of black women residents in the locality was 21.5 per cent, that of hospice service users 1 to 2 per cent, while group membership included no black women. A series of hospice initiatives was underway, such as research into referral patterns and provision for interpreters, which the facilitators hoped would begin to address the issue. However, as postmodern groupwork theorizing has highlighted, group interaction can itself constitute a further barrier to equal participation through certain discourses dominating over others (Tapping 1991). In this case, one facilitator described instances of racist innuendo in discussion. Therefore, if women from minority ethnic groups had joined, they would have been likely to experience discrimination.

This situation also underlined the importance of anti-discriminatory perspectives in augmenting a self-directed approach to groupwork. The facilitator now saw the importance of setting out more clearly the unacceptability of racist statements, when discussing a group's ground rules, as a basis for challenging them. She described worriedly how, in keeping with a self-directed approach, she had tried to proceed 'quite softly', but had become aware that 'unless we do challenge, there's going to be this kind of racist undercurrent'. The potentially key role of facilitators is highlighted here since pressure for change seemed unlikely to come from group members. When interviewed, no member spontaneously raised the absence of women from minority ethnic groups as a shortcoming in the group. Two acknowledged being 'prejudiced', one commenting: 'I suppose I shouldn't be, but you can't help the way you are. I never show it. I always treat them all right, you know.'

Heterosexism

The social work facilitator's account also revealed how the group reflected another wide trend, that of lesbian and bisexual women's interests being marginalized through the form taken by the dominant discourse (Butler and Wintram 1991). Despite the commitment in the group's information leaflet to meeting lesbian women's requirements, she described how group discussion slid into assuming that all group members were heterosexual. As a facilitator, she felt she had failed to counter this effectively. Consequently, the group contributed to perpetuating, not challenging, the marginalization of older lesbian women's interests in health care (Archibald and Baikie 1998).

The risk of emotional damage

In keeping with feminist and palliative care traditions, the group had addressed emotional needs as integral to physical well-being. Nevertheless, one member's account showed how such groups are not proof against emotional damage being incurred by women whose well-being is already under threat (Hitch *et al.* 1994). When interviewed, everyone commented on the group's friendliness. However, one member identified shortcomings. Describing herself as already very depressed, she related how she had nearly left the group because she had been so distressed by another group member berating her for self-centredness. This had occurred when the respondent had talked about thinking 'Why me?', concerning her diagnosis of SBC. The incident had gone unnoticed by remaining group members and facilitators. However, it illustrates how all parties to such groups need to be aware that members do not escape the risk of responses that are damaging to mental health needs.

A self- or facilitator-controlled group?

The problematic effects of hierarchical power relations between professional facilitators and lay group members remain an issue in feminist groupwork (Saulnier 2000). The concern is that facilitators dominating group activity stifle group members' initiative in overcoming social disadvantage.

Evidence from this group suggests that facilitator–group member power relations are more complex than this. The preceding accounts of discriminatory interaction indicate that facilitators don't necessarily exercise power over members, and that members' control does not guarantee equity. Facilitators may also grapple with external professional–member power conflicts. In common with the facilitators of other such groups (Monroe 1997), for example, this facilitator had encountered considerable resistance from professional colleagues to a facilitated self-help group as a resource. Facilitators may tilt professional–member power relations towards members' interests within a group, as here when they made social care information and services more readily available.

At the same time, this group illustrates that feminist commentators are right to argue that the role of facilitator runs the risk of acting as a brake on members' powers to tackle social disadvantage, even if the status quo is acceptable to all parties (Butler and Wintram 1991). Group members had no illusions about the social work facilitator's lead role in organizing and coordinating the group. Janet stated: 'Jenny runs it. . . . She'll go to everybody – everybody has the chance to talk. She'll turn and say, "What about the next one?"' Invoking the model of 'chairing', they described this as helpful because it ensured that the group was well organized, encouraged participation in discussion and maintained direction. Setting up the group, ensuring continuity and coordinating discussion might have imposed inappropriate demands on members' stamina and fluctuating health. However, ways need to be found for members to avoid being sidelined in a disablist way, both from initiating groups and from determining their agendas, if they are to ensure their requirements are met. The origins of C4Ward itself are positive evidence of the first point (McCartney 1995). The following account of group members taking charge of a session's agenda illustrates the second point:

> Somebody had asked about holidays and I thought 'I'll take this stuff in', and that was the week one member brought in some make-up and said, 'I was offered this pampering and somebody gave me a make-over.' She thought it would be nice to share it with the other women. So it wasn't appropriate for me to say, 'Oh, excuse me, I thought we were going to talk about holidays this time', because they'd got all the lipstick and foundation there was. They really thoroughly enjoyed it.
>
> (Social work facilitator)

Conclusion

This chapter confirms that women's experience reflects the impact of sexism on health but in interaction with further forms of social disadvantage – such as ageism, relative poverty, disablism, racism and heterosexism – interacting with each other in turn. It shows how group relations are permeated by unequal contemporary social conditions whose effects cannot be airbrushed out by concentrating on universal and timeless rules of how groups unfold. Instead, the impact of such conditions needs to be recognized in order to address them in the interests of group members' well-being. Despite these obstacles, primarily through the mutual support and enhanced knowledge and resources it can create, groupwork that incorporates a focus on gender can make a vibrant contribution to greater equality in health.

References

Addington Hall, J. and McCarthy, M. (1993) 'Dying from cancer: results of a national population-based investigation', *Palliative Medicine*, 9: 295–305.

Age Concern England (1996) *Age Concern Briefings. Breast Screening and Older Women: Statistics*, Ref. 1595, London: Age Concern England.

—— (1999) *Turning Your Back on Us*, London: Age Concern England.

Archibald, C. and Baikie, E. (1998) 'The sexual politics of old age', in Phillips, J. and Bernard, M. (eds) *The Social Policy of Old Age*, London: Centre for Policy on Ageing.

Baum, M., Saunders, C. and Meredith, S. (1995) *Breast Cancer*, Oxford: Oxford University Press.

Bernard, M. (2000) *Promoting Health in Old Age*, Milton Keynes: Open University.

Burch, R. (1997) 'Alive and Kicking', *Nursing Times*, 93, 9: 6–12.

Butler, S. and Wintram, C. (1991) *Feminist Groupwork*, London: Sage.

Bywaters, P. and McLeod, E. (eds) (1996) *Working for Equality in Health*, London: Routledge.

Cohen, M. and Mullender, A. (1999) 'The personal in the political: exploring the group work continuum from individual to social change goals', *Social Work With Groups*, 22, 1: 13–31.

Collins, W., Friedman, E. and Pivot, A. (eds) (1978) *The Directory of Social Change: Women*, London: Wildwood House.

Croft, S. (1996) 'How can I leave them? Towards an empowering social work practice with women who are dying', in Fawcett, B., Galloway, M. and Perrins, J. (eds) *Feminism and Social Work in the Year 2000*, Bradford: University of Bradford.

—— and Beresford, P. (1997)'Service users' perspectives', in Davies, M. (ed.) *The Blackwell Companion to Social Work*, Oxford: Blackwell.

Doyal, L. (1995) *What Makes Women Sick?* Basingstoke: Macmillan.

Falkingham, J. (1998) 'Financial (in)security in later life', in Bernard, M. and Phillips, J. (eds) *The Social Policy of Old Age*, London: Centre for Policy on Ageing.

Finch, J. (1982) 'A women's health group in Mansfield', in Curno, A., Lamming, A., Leach, L., Stiles, J., Ward, V., Wright, A. and Ziff, T. (eds) *Women in Collective Action*, London: Routledge & Kegan Paul.

Firth, P. (2000) 'Picking up the pieces: groupwork in palliative care', *Groupwork*, 12, 1: 27–41.

Gordon, D., Shaw, M., Dorling, D., and Davey Smith, G. (1999) *Inequalities in Health*, Bristol: Policy Press.

Gott, M., Stevens, T., Small, N., and Hjelmeland Ahmedzai, S. (2000) *User Involvement in Cancer Care*, Bristol: Policy Press.

Graham, H. (ed.) (2000) *Understanding Health Inequalities*, Buckingham: Open University Press.

Granville, G. (2000) 'Menopause: a time of private change to a mature identity', in Bernard, M., Phillips, J., Machin, L. and Harding Davies, V. (eds) *Women Ageing*, London: Routledge.

Greenwood, V. and Young, J. (1976) *Abortion on Demand*, London: Pluto Press.

Hitch, P.J., Fielding, R.G., and Llewelyn, S.P. (1994) 'Effectiveness of self-help and support groups for cancer patients: a review', *Psychology and Health*, 9: 437–48.

Littlewood, J. (1992) *Aspects of Grief*, London: Routledge.

Lockett, M. (1996) *Breast Cancer Workshop Report*, London: Channel 4 Television (available from C4Ward, Breast Cancer Care, Kiln House, 210 New Kings Road, London SW6 4NZ).

McCartney, A. (1995) *Alive and Kicking*, London: Channel 4 Television.

MacKeith, N. (ed.) (1978) *Womens' Health Handbook*, London: Virago.

McLeod, E. (1998) 'Women with secondary breast cancer: developing self-help support groups', *Practice*, 10, 3: 13–26.

McLeod, E. (2000) *Facing it Together: Older Women, Secondary Breast Cancer and Self-Help Support Groups*, Birmingham: Age Concern (available from Age Concern Birmingham, Centro House, 16 Summer Lane, Birmingham B19 3SD, UK).

McLeod, E. and Bywaters, P. (2000) *Social Work, Health and Equality*, London: Routledge.

Manor, O. (1999) 'Help as mutual aid: groupwork in mental health', *Groupwork*, 11, 3: 30–49.

Monroe, B. (1997) 'Facilitating groups for people with terminal illness', *Proceedings of the Congress of the European Association of Palliative Care*, Barcelona: European Association of Palliative Care.

National Cancer Alliance (1996) *Patient-Centred Cancer Services?* Oxford: National Cancer Alliance.

O'Connor, P. (1992) *Friendships Between Women*, Hemel Hempstead: Harvester Wheatsheaf.

Oliviere, D., Hargreaves, R., and Monroe, B. (1998) *Good Practices in Palliative Care*, Aldershot: Ashgate Arena.

Positively Women (1994) *Women Like Us*, London: Positively Women.

Saulnier, C.F. (2000) 'Incorporating feminist theory into social work practice: group work examples', *Social Work With Groups*, 23, 1: 5–29.

Tapping, C. (1991) 'Challenging the dominant story: behind the "worthy of discussion" groups', *Dulwich Centre Newsletter*, 4: 35–9 (Sydney, Australia: Dulwich Centre).

Weaver, R. (1996) 'Localities and inequalities: locality management in the inner city', in Bywaters, P. and McLeod, E. (eds) *Working for Equality in Health*, London: Routledge.

Chapter 15

Feminist group work and homelessness

David E. Pollio and Tonya Edmond

With its roots in an inequitable economic system, homelessness disproportionately affects minority populations and women, and is perpetuated by social injustice and oppression. The often politicized issues of mental illness and substance abuse further complicate it. Group workers have long recognized the challenges of working with this population. For approximately two decades, the group work literature has provided myriad examples of programs developed for and provided to homeless people. Some of the most innovative and creative applications in group practice have developed in response to meeting the needs of people who are homeless.

Group work, concerned with social experiences and issues of power, represents a natural ground for feminist practice (Johnson and Lee 1994). Many groups serving the homeless population develop models based on feminist theory and practice. Consequently, issues such as leadership and community are approached from perspectives that are substantially different from more traditional models.

The incorporation of feminist theory into practice with homeless people is particularly important given recent evidence documenting the substantial proportion of the homeless population who are women and children (Burt *et al.* 1999). The importance of the role of gender in homelessness is probably underestimated due to the number in programs not traditionally included in population counts, such as those for abused women, many of whom are at high risk of homelessness (Dail and Koshes 1992). Increased vulnerability to victimization and the general societal oppression of women complicate the task of successfully addressing the needs of this particularly important sub-set of the homeless population. Therefore, exploring the circumstances of abused women allows generalization to other homeless groups, in the conceptualization and development of feminist group work practice.

The purpose of this chapter is to review the literature on group work with homeless people from a feminist perspective. We provide an overview of the population, followed by a discussion of groups for homeless people, and then a presentation of our feminist framework for inquiry. This framework consists of features that we see as shared across feminist group practice, followed by questions relevant to addressing each feature in practice. A specific focus on abused women structured by this framework forms the fourth section.

Overview of homelessness in the USA

Defining homelessness

Describing the homeless population is in itself a political task. How one defines "homelessness" has an impact on the characteristics of the population observed and, subsequently, on the focus of policy and intervention. For example, if the term "homeless" is understood narrowly as denoting people who are literally sleeping outdoors or in shelters, those who are living in makeshift living situations, at high risk for literal homelessness, will be excluded from concern. Because this chapter is service-focused rather than descriptive, we propose a definition which would include anyone seeking or receiving either homeless services, or services aimed at individuals or families at risk for homelessness. Although we focus primarily on homelessness, many or all of our points are equally applicable to the entire population characterized by extreme poverty.

Gender differences in homelessness

It is not appropriate to discuss group work with homeless people without considering gender. Population studies (North and Smith 1992) indicate that men are more likely than women to have a substance-use or dependence diagnosis and are more likely to exhibit traits associated with antisocial personality disorder. Women are more likely than men to meet criteria for depression and, for those meeting criteria for addiction (approximately one-quarter of the population), their substance of choice is most likely to be alcohol. Additionally, homeless women are much more likely to have suffered abuse or violence, which will most typically have been inflicted by their partners. Finally, comparing the population with mental illness to those who do not meet diagnostic criteria, North and colleagues (1996) found evidence affirming the existence of a distinct "bag lady" profile – an older woman with an alcohol problem and a mental illness diagnosis.

Group constructs for homeless service provision

The literature provides a number of constructs around which discussions of group work and homelessness can be focused. Presenting these allows us to identify the additional options available through the inclusion of feminist thought into group service delivery for homeless people. In particular, our interest is in group formation and purpose, group goals, and relationships among group members.

Group formation and purpose

The first construct concerns the forces leading to group formation, as well as the initial group purpose. Often, groups described in the homelessness literature are recruited from available populations, professionally led, and have an agenda focused on individual interventions delivered in a collective setting (Berman-Rossi and Cohen 1988; Mancoske and Lindhorst 1991; Martin and Nayowith 1988). This construct is in line with traditional group work. Of central concern for these groups are composition considerations, in terms both of personalities and desired outcomes.

The research on groups and homelessness, and much of the feminist group literature, identifies potential purposes for creating groups other than for professional intervention. One example can be found in groups that come together, out of shared interests, and organize collectively (Cohen and Wagner 1992). Another example comes from Breton (1988) who describes a group that organized within a women's shelter. The group, which included both workers and service participants, formed to address a community issue of mutual concern. Issues like composition were handled within the group and the roles of group members emerged from the collective, rather than being imposed by a force external to the group, such as a service professional.

Another alternative to professional intervention is one where individuals identifying as homeless come together across a variety of service settings to promote a shared agenda. Pollio *et al.* (1996) describe an example of this type of group, in which service participants and providers organized a voter registration campaign, a candidates' forum, and transportation to the polls for a city council election held at a multi-service street center. By collectively organizing, the homeless community was able to have an impact on the individual candidates, and thus on the city's politics. This example expands the definition of group membership in that it recognizes a structure emerging from the "street community" rather than a structure being imposed by a professional setting (Pollio 1995).

Group goals

The second construct often discussed in the homelessness group work literature is related to group goals. In particular, the group literature divides this discussion into goals related to changing individuals within the group versus goals related to changing social structures. It should be noted that group goals in the context of homelessness are generally not narrowly conceived as consisting entirely of one or the other. Often, individual goals will be confounded by larger social problems. For example, becoming "housed" is impossible where there are insufficient numbers of affordable units, and the group might discuss this. Similarly, participating in a social change group can have a positive impact on an individual's self-confidence and ability to act independently.

Relationships among group members

The final construct concerns the relationships among group members. The homelessness group literature includes considerations similar to those of the general group work literature, such as process and development. In addition, this literature generally includes a strong focus on social support and relationships outside of the group.

Some researchers have described social supports for homeless people as being weak and ineffectual, often attenuating the longer a person remains homeless (Rossi *et al*. 1986; Grigsby *et al*. 1990). The ethnographic literature, as well as recent quantitative work, suggest that this characterization is simplistic. Descriptions of social groups within the homeless community abound. Examples of indigenous groups include "streetcorner groups" (Liebow 1965), "bottle gangs" (Anderson 1978), and "hang out groups" (Pollio 1994). Researchers have described a variety of social connections around survival and maintenance in street settings (Snow and Anderson 1987; Wagner 1993; Pollio 1994).

Recent research has provided evidence that membership of these groups is associated with service entry and the course of homelessness. Pollio (1999) found that location and the presence of a self-identified group acted as either a risk or a protective factor for service use, depending on the location of the group. Eyrich *et al*. (2001) developed and tested a substitution hypothesis in examining social supports. They found that, as non-homeless ties decreased, networks of similar size and support within homeless environments replaced them. The conclusion of this recent research has important implications for discussing group practice with this population. It suggests the presence and impact of existing social networks or groups on homeless behavior. It further implies that it is important to recognize the omnipresence and significance of such naturally occurring social support groups as an integral part of any discussion of group work with homeless people.

A feminist framework for inquiry

In this section we present features commonly found in the feminist practice literature. We believe that feminist group work with homeless people exhibits the following:

- genuine power sharing among group members;
- the exploration of personal behaviors as having political meaning;
- a focus on community identity and on individual empowerment; and
- an understanding of the group's purpose as both therapeutic and community change-oriented.

Genuine power sharing among all group members

A good opening question for feminist group workers is "Have I genuinely provided a structure in which all group members share power?" This position differs from related practice modalities, such as strength-based approaches, in that it moves beyond recognizing the positives that service participants bring to interventions to ensuring that the members share their strengths with one another through the group's power structure. Support for this is provided in Cohen's discussion (1994) of leadership among homeless adults.

The commitment to genuine power sharing has important ramifications for group leadership by professional service providers. First, it requires self-awareness on the part of leaders to ensure that they have not assumed any of the traditional power trappings around group leadership. This includes issues such as member recruitment and group composition, and roles within individual sessions and across the life span of the group. Assuming a more open stance on membership and structure requires questioning many traditional group work assumptions around leadership.

Cohen, in her 1998 article on power relationships, presents an important challenge to the concept of genuine power sharing. She argues that social work may be unable to fully realize this, given the field's hierarchical nature. It may be true that the privilege inherent in professional status may inhibit full power sharing. There is a clear power imbalance between a housed professional social worker and an unemployed homeless person. Nonetheless, the goal should be pursued to the fullest extent possible.

Power sharing does not require a social worker to relinquish a facilitative role within the group. It is generally the case that the professional has unique strengths and insights of his/her own. Sharing power does not mean disowning knowledge and expertise; rather it means valuing it for *all* group members. It means providing information, expertise and self in such a manner that the group is empowered to make informed choices. Although group recruitment and within-group structures might resemble those of traditional models, when the group is empowered to make its own determinations with regard to these issues power is shared within the group.

Assuring that power is *meaningfully* shared in developing and recruiting groups is, however, often limited to the initial phase of group development. In order to truly incorporate power sharing into group work, we must focus both on how this state is achieved and on how it is maintained over the life of the group. We must understand how power sharing emerges in the group process as well as the experiences that lead to the identification of various levels of expertise for group members. We must continue to explore opportunities to increase power sharing as the group becomes more intimate. Further, power must be examined and understood as it emerges within the dynamics among group members as they develop over time. Finally, power must be continually examined as the group relates to outside power structures, such as the agency or the broader social and political environment.

Examining personal behaviors as having political meaning

In discussing mainstream feminism, the idea that the personal is also the political is almost axiomatic. If anything, for the homeless population this feature of feminism is even more important. Feminist group work practitioners need to be cognizant of:

- the public nature of the lives of homeless persons and how their every action is available for examination;
- the interpretation of individuals' actions, whether as negative stereotype or positive action against oppression;
- the importance of one's own actions towards persons who are homeless; and
- the unique meaning of everyday interactions with social institutions.

Persons who are obviously homeless are often victims of stereotypes about all homeless people. Research has found that they themselves are acutely aware of this. A story told by a homeless person illustrates this aptly:

> One time, I was sitting across the street . . . and this other [homeless] guy sat down and said [to this business man] "Excuse me sir." He said [the business man] "I ain't got no change," and he [the homeless person] said "No, I just wanted to know the time . . . you already pre-judged."
>
> (Pollio and Kasden 1996: 118)

Social action, initiated or driven by homeless individuals themselves, has the potential for added political force. This may be attributed to the breaking of prevailing stereotypes (e.g. "I didn't know those bums could act for themselves") or more noble sentiments (e.g. "Look at those victims of oppression fighting in spite of the obstacles"). In either case, when a particular population acts for itself in a way that appears to the larger society as atypical, the political meaning of their actions, and often the impact of those actions, are increased.

Yet another instance of personal action having political meaning can be seen in the change of attitudes of service providers towards persons who are homeless. The literature is filled with examples of providers who have had their attitudes changed by persons who are homeless (see e.g. Cohen and Johnson 1997). Many examples describe service providers who have had to re-evaluate their attitudes towards homelessness and homeless individuals (e.g. Pollio and Kasden 1996). Both altered public attitudes towards homeless persons by service providers and change effected by challenging hierarchical attitudes represent separate applications of this concept.

One last application of feminist theory as it relates to the political meaning of personal behavior can be found in the interaction between homeless persons and larger social institutions. A prosaic example of interaction that is imbued with additional political meaning would be the relationship between being homeless and receiving mail. Public entitlements generally require a mailing address for both receipt and completion of additional forms. So both the application for and receipt of many benefits are made substantially more difficult for a person with no address. For this reason, and many others, establishing an address becomes critically important. Further, when agencies have established mail addresses for their clients, the act has taken on a meaning beyond simply creating a place to receive benefits.

It establishes a location grounded in a community and a collective identity, one leading to increased political power and potential for collective action.

Focusing on community identity and individual empowerment

We have already emphasized the importance of social ties among the homeless community. Reports from group practice with the homeless population have revealed that an emerging community identity is related to achieving individual change (Breton 1988; Glasser and Suroviak 1988; Pollio 1990, 1994). Brown and Zeifort (1990) have argued that, for women, reconnecting with community is a critical stage in exiting homelessness.

Johnson and Lee, in their 1994 article on empowerment and feminist practice with women who are homeless, emphasize the bonds that connect women in oppressed situations and their potential utility for practice. We agree strongly with this observation, and would broaden its applicability by suggesting that it is important to recognize the bonds that connect all homeless people (Pollio 1999). Professional intervention in general, and group work specifically, must construct itself within the shared experience and social construct of homelessness.

Up to this point, we have conceptualized "community" only in the broadest sense, positing a generic existence and shared characteristics among the homeless population. In focusing on the utility of community identity in a way that is relevant to practice, it is necessary for the practitioner to deconstruct "community identity" further.

First, community boundaries need to be understood for the specific geographic location. What constitutes the "edge" of the community? Is it the city, the neighborhood, or some other geographic feature, such as a social center location? Second, it is also necessary to examine who is considered to be within the community and who is deemed to fall outside it. This is particularly important in understanding the relationship of the service provider to the community. For example, Pollio (1994) discussed his own relationship with a specific group of homeless people and how he gradually moved from outside the group towards membership. His relationship with the group changed throughout this process as he gradually achieved inclusion. Third, "community" may be understood by what it affords homeless persons in their daily task of surviving. By that standard, "community" might be defined by the interrelationships within the individual service system. An example of that form of deconstruction might ask: which shelters are connected to which food kitchens, which clothing closets (places that distribute donated clothing free of charge) and service centers? Conceptually, depending on the structure of the service system, multiple interrelated communities may exist within single boundaries.

In conducting feminist inquiry that informs practice, we must reconstruct our community using at least one, and likely more, of these layered constructs. Beyond allowing the communities a voice in guiding our reconstruction, we must also continue our exploration of the social construction and meaning of these communities in our practice. Further, we must inquire beyond the obvious deficits typically emphasized in order to identify the strengths of, and the possibilities for empowering, homeless persons.

Understanding group purpose as both therapeutic and community change-oriented

In our discussion of group constructs (pp. 178–80), we emphasized the group's potential for having goals related to both personal growth and social change. What lends this assertion particular value for our inquiry is the impact that it has on our understanding of group processes.

Rather than seeing group process as consisting entirely of either individual goals, with personal interactions as the mechanism for individual change, or instrumental goals achieved by focusing on social content, we follow Cohen and Mullender's assertion (1999) that group process can include multiple non-exclusive features of individual change, personal interactions, and impact on social environment. Further, we would sub-divide interpersonal content into instrumental and support aspects. Thus, the interpersonal interaction among group members provides not only solutions to the problems facing homeless individuals, but also the support and connectedness of sharing their personal difficulties.

In focusing on how this might guide feminist inquiry, we end up facing in two directions – inward towards the group and outward towards the social environment in which the group resides. In looking inward, we assert that our inquiry must focus on how the individual, the interpersonal (both instrumentally and through support), and the social interact within the group's process. Nevertheless, it has repeatedly been observed that it is impossible for an individual to become housed, irrespective of how high the desire for change is, unless appropriate affordable housing is available (cf. Burt 1991). In this situation, individual change is not the appropriate goal – social change is. Additionally, since it has been reported that becoming housed has a mediating effect on mental illness (North *et al.* 1998), we would contend that social action has the potential added benefit of addressing an individual-level issue.

Thus, inquiry must first be made to determine the possibilities for direct first-order changes. In other words, the group process must determine its ability to directly promote change for individuals and/or society. Next, it is necessary to examine the group's potential to create second-order changes. Social change may have a secondary, indirect impact on the group through individual-level outcomes. Conversely, individual change, through developing and instilling a sense of empowerment within members, may have secondary impact by promoting an individual's group participation, thus motivating social action.

Because it is not possible to identify at once all of the potential for change within a group, the interrelationship between levels of change must also continue to be addressed over the life of the group. Changes at tertiary levels (social change, prompting individual change, prompting further social action), and beyond, must continue to be explained.

Abused women and homelessness

In this section, we focus on abused women and the group-based models suggested by the framework developed above. We begin with the context within which abused women become homeless and the obstacles they face in their attempts to exit homelessness.

The exigencies of being a victim of violence can directly increase the likelihood of becoming homeless. For example, one avenue through which people become homeless is by having to leave the temporary shelter of family or friends. For an abused woman, this already difficult situation is often exacerbated by the threat of physical violence posed by her abuser toward anyone who protects her. Similarly, abused women often encounter employment difficulties, such as loss of jobs as a result of their abusers harassing them on the phone, verbally or physically assaulting them on the job, or simply preventing them from making it to work. Some women, having never been allowed by their abuser to work, face the challenges of finding employment with little or no experience in the workplace.

The lack of transitional housing, affordable permanent housing, and childcare makes an abused woman's situation all the more precarious. In many communities, the waiting list for resources can range from a few months to several years. The deep cuts in our welfare system have resulted in such severe restrictions and limitations that, even with full benefits, it is often impossible for the woman to maintain housing. This level of economic vulnerability is a primary reason why abused women often feel compelled to return to the abuser. In addition to the severe financial stress of the situation, woman abuse also inflicts an enormous psychological toll, frequently leading to depression, anxiety and post-traumatic stress disorder. These additional factors compound the difficulties of the situation and further increase abused women's vulnerability to becoming homeless.

Many abused women, in an effort to cope with the overwhelming trauma they are experiencing, resort to alcohol and/or other substance abuse, a response that has the unfortunate consequence of increasing the risks of subsequent victimization (Miller *et al.* 1989; Miller *et al.* 1993), as well as adding to the vulnerabilities associated with homelessness. Further, many shelters (refuges) deny admission to substance-abusing women and most substance abuse programs ignore the role of violence against women in the development of such disorders. Additionally, there are too few treatment programs available that provide childcare or allow children to stay with their mothers in residential settings. Some abused women are thus faced with the dilemma of having to place their children in temporary care in order to get help. Unfortunately, it can be a slow and arduous process trying to get the children back, a process that has resulted in many becoming wards of the state, which ironically is a risk factor for their eventually becoming homeless (Simons and Whitbeck 1991).

It is because of these social injustices that feminist group work practice plays such an important role in work with homeless abused women. The question then becomes "What does feminist group work with homeless abused women look like?" To answer that question, we return to the framework presented previously.

Genuine power sharing among the group members

From the beginning, feminists working in the movement to end violence against women have challenged the traditional structure of group work, particularly with respect to power and authority. This challenging philosophical perspective, when held by a group facilitator, enhances power sharing among group members. Inherent in this position is the critical notion that abused women are experts on their own lives, rather than that all expertise resides with the group leader. We have found in our work that it is beneficial to acknowledge overtly the expertise we recognize in each woman and to express our desire to learn from her. This can be a significant approach to power sharing, providing it is done from a standpoint of genuineness. It communicates a respect and a mutuality that can reduce hierarchy and enhance power sharing.

When power is shared in this manner, members learn that they have something of value to contribute to each other and to the group leader. Recognizing that they have something to give the group often makes it easier for women to believe that they deserve to receive the support and assistance that are being offered. Through this process of exchange, leadership moves around the group members, rather than being held by the designated (professional) leader. As a consequence, the unique knowledge, skills, and interpersonal talents that individual group members possess are called forth and become engaged as they work together to address the issues that unfold within the group context.

This type of group process involves a less formal approach to interactions between group leader and group members. In many respects, the group leader operates more as a group facilitator than a group expert. The substantial differences between the status accorded on the one hand to a social worker and on the other to a homeless abused woman necessitate the use of such an approach if rapport and trust are to be established and maintained, and if power sharing is to be maximized. Ideally, participation in a group is voluntary and the members are engaged in the process of forming and defining the group structure. For example, members should have a voice in the development of group guidelines around confidentiality, meeting times, topics to be discussed, the degree to which one participates in discussions, and termination.

Examining personal behaviors as having political meaning

The very personal and painful experiences that homeless abused women go through have political meaning because those violent and oppressive acts are embedded in our social institutions and are often sanctioned by our governmental policies, such as welfare "reform." This has increased the barriers in the way of women leaving their abusers by greatly reducing the availability of benefits for single parents. Feminist group work practitioners bring their understanding of this structural analysis, a critical component of their intervention, to the attention of the homeless abused women with whom they work, thereby deepening their awareness of those factors and facilitating their empowerment.

For abused women, the public acknowledgment of their victimization carries the potential for both stigma and survival. The act of leaving an abusive relationship has the potential to be an act of great political consequence: the public affirmation of refusing to accept the role of victim. It also carries with it the risk of perpetuating negative stereotypes. For abused women who have to temporarily relinquish child custody because of inadequate shelter options, being homeless carries the additional likelihood of being negatively labeled.

In terms of practice, this latter example carries the potential to reinterpret the negative stereotype as a positive action against oppression, both for the victim and for the observing (and frequently hostile) outside community. Refusing to accept our own stereotypes, and carefully considering our actions jointly with the victim of abuse, gives political meaning to the oppression of the individual who is forced to relinquish her children as a result of a social inadequacy (lack of support for families). Additionally, our own actions in refusing to accept the negative stereotype adds a potent statement of our own to this political meaning.

Focus on community identity and empowerment

It is tragically ironic that, given the astonishing prevalence of violence against women, the experience of victimization leaves the woman feeling profoundly isolated. It was through breaking the silence around domestic violence and sexual assault that women discovered they were not alone. In the act of breaking the silence, a community was formed, dedicated to ending violence against women.

The commonality of our vulnerability to exploitation and to various forms of violence created a connection among women, a shared understanding of what it means to be female in a sexist culture. Thus, community has been a central feature of feminist practice within the movement to end violence against women. Its essence is captured in the well-known notion of sisterhood and is reflected in the recognition that, by virtue of our gender, we are all at risk and thus must all support one another in our struggle to end violence and oppression in our lives.

Yet there are many layers to what constitutes "community," and feminist group practitioners must recognize these communities of interest as defined by the group members. Those that are significant to abused homeless women may be defined as family and friends, other homeless persons, and members of an ethnic or cultural group, to name a few. Furthermore, what initially constitutes "community" for a group member may evolve and change over time as the group progresses. The practitioner should expect that as groups coalesce a sense of community is experienced. Thus, a homeless abused woman may come into group having never before disclosed her experiences of being sexually or physically abused and, in breaking the silence, may realize that she is not alone and for the first time have a sense of identification with other survivors.

It is important for feminist group work practitioners to recognize that abusers will have systematically isolated abused women from almost all sense and sources of community. Thus, reconnection is not just an initial phase in the development of the group, but an important source of healing and empowerment to its members. A feminist group practitioner should be cognizant of the significance of the various communities and should help the group members identify the sources of support as well as of stress that are exchanged between them, examine the resources available within each of those sources, and identify ways to initiate and/or strengthen connections to them. In reconnecting with community, homeless abused women are empowered to reclaim their sense of self and of identity.

Understanding group purpose as being both therapeutic and community change-oriented

Given the structural inequalities within our culture that facilitate both homelessness and violence against women, as social workers and feminist practitioners we must select interventions that target community change. One could argue, however, that we have an equally compelling reason to select interventions that facilitate the healing of the damage to the individual inflicted by violence and oppression. Feminist group work is one of the few interventionist options available: one that not only allows, but actually encourages, the pursuit of both goals simultaneously. In working on individual-level changes with homeless abused women, it is essential that the feminist group worker be aware of the risks of inadvertently engaging in, and thereby reinforcing, victim blaming within and between group members. This is particularly important, since we live in a society that typically views problems such as abuse, homelessness, and substance abuse as being attributable to individual deficits. It must be made explicitly clear to group members that abused women are not responsible for the violence they have experienced or for the homelessness that may ensue as a result of that abuse. It is also important to acknowledge the social context within which substance abuse occurs.

Abused women deserve a safe place to process the multiple traumas they have experienced without their symptoms of distress being used against them. In fact, an important task for the group leader is to provide the members with educational information about the dynamics of abuse, gender inequality and issues of power and control, as well as how trauma is processed. This psycho-educational approach can be very empowering for abused women and can effectively dispel victim-blaming myths that they may have internalized. In addition to providing such information, it is also important and empowering for the group worker to facilitate the development of safety plans with each group member.

Because feminist group work practitioners have an understanding of the structural analysis of the factors behind violence against women and homelessness, attention to individual change is both therapeutic and empowering. It occurs within the mutually supportive personal interactions among group members who can collectively become a powerful voice in advocating for community change. Thus, by helping group members to understand the processes that contributed to their current situation and to identify the external sources in the system in which they live, we assist individuals towards changing those systems. Many examples of such change efforts exist throughout diverse social movements, and such efforts should be encouraged and facilitated by feminist group work practitioners.

Toward the future of feminist group practice

We have begun a dialog on how feminist group work might be conceptualized for homeless populations, particularly for women. We hope that this presentation of ideas represents only a starting place for practitioners, policy makers, researchers, and our homeless partners. We encourage readers to incorporate into this dialog additional levels of complexity brought through integrating other topics discussed within this book, as these interface with issues raised here.

We end this chapter with a challenge to practitioners and researchers to take our ideas as a starting place for attention to feminist practice and group work with the homeless population. A shared observation for us across our practice and research careers has been the cogent voice brought to our thinking by persons who are homeless. We further challenge readers to include individuals who are homeless in their own work, confident that this will bring on-going attention to a major experience of oppression and social injustice.

References

Anderson, E. (1978) *A Place on the Corner*, Chicago, IL: University of Chicago Press.

Berman-Rossi, T. and Cohen, M.B. (1988) "Group development and shared decision making: working with homeless mentally ill women," *Social Work With Groups*, 11, 4: 63–78.

Breton, M. (1988) "The need for mutual aid groups in a drop-in center for homeless women: the sistering case," *Social Work With Groups*, 11, 4: 47–61.

Brown, K.S. and Zeifort, M. (1990) "A feminist approach to working with homeless women," *Affilia*, 5, 1: 6–20.

Burt, M. (1991) *Over the Edge: The Growth of Homelessness in the 1980s*, New York: Russell Sage.

Burt, M., Douglass, T., Valente, J., Lee, E., and Iwen, B. (1999) *Homelessness: Programs and the Persons they Serve. Findings of the National Survey of Homeless Assistance Providers and Clients*, Washington, DC: Bureau of the Census.

Cohen, M.B. (1994) "Who wants to chair the meeting? Group development and leadership patterns in a community action group of homeless people," *Social Work*, 39, 6: 742–9.

Cohen, M.B. (1998) "Perceptions of power in client/worker relationships," *Families in Society*, 79, 4: 433–42.

Cohen, M.B. and Johnson, J. (1997) "Poetry in motion: a self-directed community group for homeless people," in Gill, J. and Parry, J. (eds) *From Prevention to Wellness Through Group Work*, New York: Haworth Press: 131–42.

Cohen, M.B. and Mullender, A. (1999) "The personal in the political: exploring the group work continuum from individual to social change goals," *Social Work With Groups*, 22, 1: 13–31.

Cohen, M.B. and Wagner, D. (1992) "Acting on their own behalf: affiliation and political mobilization among homeless people," *Journal of Sociology and Social Welfare*, 19, 4: 21–39.

Dail, P.W. and Koshes, R.J. (1992) "Treatment issues and treatment configurations for mentally ill homeless women," *Social Work in Health Care*, 17, 4: 27–44.

Eyrich, K.M., Pollio, D.E. and North, C.S. (2001) "Differences in social support between short-term and long-term homelessness," unpublished manuscript.

Glasser, I. and Suroviak, J. (1988) "Social group work in a soup kitchen: mobilizing the strengths of the guests", *Social Work With Groups*, 11, 4: 95–109.

Grigsby, C., Baumann, D., Gregorich, S.E. and Roberts-Gray, C. (1990) "Dissafiliation to entrenchment: a model for understanding homelessness," *Journal of Social Issues*, 46, 4: 141–56.

Johnson, A.J. and Lee, J.A.B. (1994) "Empowerment work with homeless women," in Mirkin, M. (ed.) *Women in Context: Toward a Feminist Reconstruction of Psychotherapy*, New York: Guilford Press.

Liebow, E. (1965) *Tally's Corner*, Boston, MA: Little, Brown and Co.

Mancoske, R.J. and Lindhorst, T. (1991) "Mutual assistance groups in a shelter for persons with AIDS," *Social Work With Groups*, 14, 2: 75–86.

Martin, M.A. and Nayowith, S. (1988) "Creating community: group work to develop social networks with homeless mentally ill," *Social Work With Groups*, 11, 4: 79–93.

Miller, B.A., Downs, W.R. and Gondoli, D.M. (1989) "Spousal violence among alcoholic women as compared to a random household sample of women," *Journal of Studies on Alcohol*, 30, 6: 533–40.

Miller, B.A., Downs, W.R. and Testa, M. (1993) "Interrelationships between victimization experiences and women's alcohol use", *Journal of Studies on Alcohol*, Supplement 11, September: 109–117.

North, C.S., Pollio, D.E., Thompson, S., Smith, E.M. and Spitznagel, E.L. (1998) "The association of psychiatric diagnosis with weather conditions in a large urban homeless sample," *Social Psychiatry and Psychiatric Epidemiology*, 33, 5: 206–11.

North, C.S. and Smith, E.M. (1992) "A systematic study of mental health services' utilization by homeless men and women," *Social Psychiatry and Psychiatric Epidemiology*, 28, 2: 77–83.

North, C.S., Smith, E.M., Pollio, D.E., and Spitznagel, E.L. (1996) "Are the mentally ill a distinct homeless subgroup?" *Annals of Clinical Psychiatry*, 8, 3: 117–28.

Pollio, D.E. (1990) "The street person: an integrated service provision model," *Psychosocial Rehabilitation Journal*, 14, 2: 57–69.

—— (1994) "Wintering at the Earle: group structures in the street community," *Social Work With Groups*, 17, 1, 2: 47–70.

—— (1995) "Hoops group: group work with persons on the streets," *Social Work With Groups*, 18, 2–3: 107–22.

—— (1999) "Group membership as a predictor of service use related behavior for persons on the streets," *Research on Social Work Practice*, 9, 5: 575–92.

Pollio, D.E. and Kasden, A. (1996) "Walking around with a question mark on your head:

social and personal constructs among persons on the streets," *Journal of Applied Social Science*, 20, 2: 107–19.

Pollio, D.E., McDonald, S.M., and North, C.S. (1996) "Combining strengths-based and feminist group work with the homeless," *Social Work With Groups*, 19, 3–4: 5–20.

Rossi, P., Fischer, G., and Willis, G. (1986) *The Condition of the Homeless in Chicago*, Amherst: Social and Demographic Research Institute, University of Massachusetts.

Simons, R.L. and Whitbeck, L.B. (1991) "Running away adolescents as a precursor to adult homelessness," *Social Service Review*, 65, 2: 224–47.

Snow, D. and Anderson, L. (1987) "Identity work among the homeless: the verbal construction and avowal of personal identities," *American Journal of Sociology*, 92, 6: 1336–71.

Wagner, D. (1993) *Checkerboard Square: Culture and Resistance in a Homeless Community*, Boulder, CO: Westview Press.

Chapter 16

Conclusion: where does this leave us?

Audrey Mullender

The postmodernist challenge: what response?

The challenges posed in Chapter 1 of this book revolved around the extent to which groupwork with a gendered content can meet the postmodernist, poststructuralist challenge of rethinking who is included within, or excluded from, traditional groupings of men and of women and whether it can move away from an essentialist polarization between the sexes towards an understanding of graduated and multiple subjectivities across a wide continuum of gender identity. Feminist groupwork in social work was arguably never the sole enclave of white, middle-class, able-bodied, affluent, heterosexual women (Butler and Wintram 1991), as the early consciousness-raising groups of the women's liberation movement were accused of being, but we should not be complacent. Thiara (Chapter 4), and also Lewis and Gutiérrez (Chapter 11), show us that minority ethnic women – including their particular examples of South Asian women in the UK and Mexican American women in the USA – have had to fight their own struggles and have not felt a part of dominant feminist discourses. Women's groups and men's groups could be seen as having been heavily grounded in universalist and sometimes simplistic notions of the pursuit of a common social justice in the face of collectively shared (or perpetrated) patriarchal oppression, so a second challenge is to recognize individual agency and goals within even the most marginalized and excluded life circumstances, and not to make women sound hopeless victims or men unchangeable aggressors or to ignore when it is women who abuse their power. Though abuse and violence remain a problem in contemporary society, and continue to be predominantly perpetrated by men, they are not women's destiny, they do not have to be tolerated, and they can be – and are – resisted in myriad seen and unseen ways. Numerous other social problems, such as ageing (see Chapter 13, by Dooley and Cox), homelessness (Chapter 15, by Pollio and Edmond), poverty (both the foregoing, and Chapter 10, by the Women First group, in view of the discrimination in employment and benefits that disabled people experience) and health status (Chapter 14, by McLeod), are gendered in their patterns and impacts so pose a similar need to think in complex non-essentialist and 'bottom–up' ways. And, like feminism, the social model of disability, which underpinned the Women First group, could be seen as another 'grand theory' pursuing social justice which has been challenged by postmodernism but which can be thought about in new, non-essentialist ways.

Beyond this, we need to consider what this anthology has had to say about gender in groupwork, particularly in terms of process, and what might be its wider messages.

Who are women and men? Engaging with diversity and difference

All the groups offered as examples in this volume have engaged with diversity and difference within gender at some level, and often in complex and unexpected ways. Just how far we have moved from a dichotomized or polarized view of gender is apparent in DeLois's chapter (9) on a group for gay, lesbian, bisexual, transsexual and questioning young people. Not only does it present a long continuum, embracing all these groupings/categories, as opposed to two stereotyped sex role opposites, but it demonstrates that people may move from point to point on the continuum over the life course, and particularly at the time in their life when they are doing the most thinking about their sexuality. Lewis and Gutiérrez (Chapter 11) also regard it as necessary to work out with potential group participants how they define gender, including their own, and what importance it currently has for them, since it is no longer acceptable to look at people and simply decide that they are male or female and that, from this, we can determine everything else about them.

Even within all-women groups, contributors have uncovered enormous diversity. The population of 'older women', for example, in Chapter 13, by Dooley and Cox, is shown to encompass women from a range of social and ethnic backgrounds, with a wide variety of abilities and health statuses, sexual orientations and marital/family situations – not surprisingly since we are talking about well over half the older population. The group for women with and without learning disabilities, in Chapter 10, by the members of Women First, worked at learning to welcome and celebrate all women rather than feeling sorry for 'grannies' or those who could not walk or talk. There was a growing recognition that valuing ourselves means valuing others, and that experiencing the world through multiple subjectivities does not obviate the need to challenge racism or to learn about diverse, non-abusive sexual preferences. Within the range of disabilities, women who do not use language, particularly if they do not communicate through any other formalized system of written or gestured signs but through noises or other more private language, are particularly discriminated against. They would almost certainly be unable to bring a court case in the UK, for example, and even service delivery decisions in social work and social care are far more likely to be imposed upon them. The Women First group pushed at the boundaries of inclusiveness in ways that are rarely matched by the official rhetoric of user involvement. This book says less about religion as a social division than might have been the case if the chapters had been drafted after 11 September 2001, when Islamophobia took on new proportions in much of the Western world, though DeLois does refer to religion intersecting, to use Lewis and Gutiérrez's term, alongside class, ethnicity, age and ability, with her central focus of interest which is sexual orientation.

McLeod's chapter (14) shows that there is diversity even within sub-groups of sub-groups of sub-groups; in this case, members who are not just all women, but older women, with health needs, and whose health needs all relate to suffering from cancer. Even with that degree of commonality, the group McLeod researched came to be formed because its founder member, having advanced secondary breast cancer, did not feel she was benefiting from meeting together with women who were expecting to get well. Her needs and issues were quite different from theirs. And even then, within the group she established, all of whose members shared similar illness experiences and who were described as 'older women', there was a twenty-one-year age span – a generation. But there was sufficient shared experience in relation to the course of the illness, the treatments used, the gaps in social and health care, and the struggles with ageism (one woman was told that she should expect pain at her age) and disablism (mobility and access barriers) to make the group a success. The need to think about multiple subjectivities, not always as overlapping experiences of discrimination but sometimes as perpetrating them, emerges from this same group where there were racist undertones, assumptions of heterosexuality and a failure to pick up on one woman's feelings of depression. Chapter 14 also draws out the differences between groupworkers and members, for example in terms of class and professional interests, as does the chapter by the Members of Women First.

Groupworkers need to see the differences as well as the commonalities between women and they need to think about which bits of themselves group members will identify with. An individual cannot split herself up and be female in one group today and black in another one tomorrow. She is female *and* black all the time. She may also be disabled and/or lesbian. Lewis and Gutiérrez describe a project in which the permutations among the staff, who, between them, had multiple social group memberships, were used to facilitate a widening range of groups. For women, multiple subjectivities affect how they can find commonality and benefit from a group. Pease (Chapter 5) and Williams (Chapter 7) show how the social divisions between men, including those of ethnicity, sexuality, class, disability and age, affect the degree to which men are able to derive privilege and power from their sex roles in society. Here, groups need enough shared experience to help the men identify with one another and also to challenge each other's sexist attitudes and behaviour.

Groupworkers need to think hard about the gender implications in all groups, whether for women or for men, or both. The example of Paul/Paula in DeLois's chapter shows that we may not even know how many men or women, or how many living in a male or female sexuality, are in the group. The gender composition of that group changed over time, though its membership did not. Being inclusive, then, is wider even than many of us may have thought, until now. As DeLois argues in relation to gay, lesbian, bisexual and transsexual people, 'We are no more monolithic than any other segment of the population but often our diversity and differences are overlooked for the sake of political unity or simplicity' (pp. 108–9). Their commonality resides largely in the shared experience of homophobia and heterosexism – in being 'othered' by a dominant sexual mores – yet there are enormous differences between radical separatist lesbians and high-camp gay men, for example. Indeed, it is heterosexuality that might be seen as occupying a narrow middle ground on a very long continuum of sexual possibilities. Similarly, in Thiara's chapter, we read about a range of groupings which, in Britain, are all lumped together as 'Asian' but which originate from vastly different religious and cultural backgrounds (urban and rural lives, for example), and from nations that have fought long and bloody wars against one another and remain at loggerheads today. South Asian women share the experience of migration to England (themselves or their families) and of experiencing racism here, but arguably little else. It is therefore not essentialist to work from commonality, as long as diversity is also recognized within it. It resides in the shared struggle to reject rigid gender roles or racial stereotypes and to challenge our understanding of them as social categories, not in defining all gay, lesbian, bi and trans people or all South Asian people – any more than all women – as somehow the same.

Challenging dichotomy

Loosley and Mullender (Chapter 8) bring the issue of dichotomy to life by challenging children's ideas about who does certain jobs in society and what they are called, and by teaching group members the concept of gender neutral language (except when naming woman abuse) in a natural and non-threatening way. The exercise used called 'Act Like a Man'/'Be Ladylike' deliberately asks young people to call forth and discuss stereotyped behaviours in males and females, and the names people are called if they step outside these. Thus socialization in the family context into polarized ideas of gender-appropriate behaviour is safely challenged in the group. In DeLois's group, participants are all now living their lives completely outside these polarized gender expectations and are learning to take pride and pleasure in who they really are. It is a joy to read about, but we know they are also still experiencing pain as a result of discrimination in the family, community and wider society.

Pease argues that the traditional and relational models of group development should not be dichotomized since, for example, profeminist men's groups might more appropriately work to the latter than to the former. In other words, we should not take an essentialist view of men's or women's experiences in groups. Gray and Healy (Chapter 12) also demonstrate that the relational model might have a useful place in mixed groups. Thus there is still some way to go in exploring what kind of continuum of groups might exist and which models might be most helpful for which group members. Pease suggests that it depends on context, objectives and ideology, not simply the sex of the members.

Hearing the silenced voices that challenge dominant discourses

For those who are doubly or multiply excluded and silenced, such as the older women in Dooley and Cox's chapter, the group takes on added importance in giving them a voice and a chance to work out what they want to say. Dominant discourses have told them that they are less worthy and should give way to men and to younger people. Telling their own story in the group, from their own perspective, casts a different light on the meaning of events and relationships in their lives. Groupwork is a particularly effective means of learning to speak out in this way because it is a supported environment where everyone is questioning what has gone before and where there is an audience to help individuals make sense of what they are newly discovering and re-evaluating about themselves.

As DeLois ably demonstrates, these dominant discourses are based in enforcement, not in anything resembling 'knowledge' or 'truth'. For example, it is the dominant heterosexual discourse that pretends there is a simple dichotomy between the straight majority and those who are deemed to be 'other'. Yet, in fact, the differences between people with diverse gay, lesbian, bisexual and transsexual orientations are so enormous that DeLois reflects 'it's sometimes hard to make the connection' (p. 109). It is important to remember, too, how far those dominant ideas have been, and still need to be, challenged. DeLois talks about Paul/Paula not having 'a diagnosable condition', but there are still medical settings in which (s)he would be 'treated' rather than empowered to discover and decide who (s)he is. In the UK, where social care is rapidly losing ground to health-care agendas, we must fight hard to hold on to social models of understanding. And, in the eyes of the law, an individual in the UK retains the sex on her/his birth certificate throughout life, even though we know that people are born emotionally trans-gendered and with a wide range of intermediate physical conditions. Our lives are thus controlled by discourses that do not even make sense and which need to be resisted and challenged at a personal or school level.

There is a connection between commonality and diversity and being able to find a voice. If we assume commonality and fail to recognize the multiple subjectivities of a group member – if, for example, there is only one young person with a direct experience of sexual abuse in a group of child witnesses of woman abuse – then he or she may continue to feel silenced, even within the group, because (s)he is 'different' from all the others. Gray and Healy, and McLeod, give examples of a single member being visibly or invisibly different from the others: the lone male in the group or the sole person who is currently depressed.

The members of some groups, such as the domestic violence perpetrators about whom Neil Blacklock writes (Chapter 6), have not been silenced but have represented the dominant discourse in their own homes, imposing their views on partners and children. The way such men talk about and understand relationships, the family and their place in it, has to be firmly confronted, but this is made the more difficult because they are in tune with, not out of sync with, the traditional and persistent treatment of women in the media, the criminal justice system, and elsewhere. Interestingly, their partners and children are the silenced voices, not only in the home but also working through into the group, where the men do not initially consider the impact of their actions on others and where it is often female groupworkers who bring these other perspectives into play. Even here, there is an interaction between being excluded and excluding others. Where abusive men simultaneously hold devalued social roles, Oliver Williams asks us to consider whether, at the same time as being challenged to exert less power in the home, black male perpetrators of domestic violence also need the group as a place where they can share experiences of being silenced, 'othered' and mistreated by white men in the workplace, the local community and the wider society. The balance for the groupworker is to hold the tension between listening to what has been silenced in the man, while never losing sight of the arenas in which he silences and abuses others.

Analysis of power: resistance and individual agency

Dooley and Cox show that older women have 'great strength, incredible resilience and social contribution' (p. 154) to offer. They are using their social agency to resist age discrimination, as they have done with sexism all their lives. In this strengths-based account, we see: power as something that can be used and attained by all; groupworkers as able to help older women gain 'a sense of their own power' (p. 156); and 'transformational practice' as the context of changes in the nature of power as well as the way it is distributed. At the other end of the age continuum, Loosley and Mullender's example of young school students working out a way to deal with inappropriate gender stereotyping by a teacher also indicates that having and using social agency does not depend on being the most powerful person in the situation. This is something to celebrate, as is Pollio and Edmond's assertion of the social agency of homeless people who have for so long been written off as derelicts and drop-outs. Michelle, in DeLois's chapter on YouthPride, says: 'I like feeling like I have some power to make the world a better place' (p. 114).

There are many ways to resist and to seek change which are open to being discussed in a group and pursued through group activity or beyond. In the chapter by the Members of Women First, there is tremendous power-sharing across what, traditionally, would be worker–member boundaries in the group. Their comment that 'we were only experts on ourselves' (p. 118) is an excellent example of making a strength out of fragmented subjectivities and challenges the assumed power of the professional, based on pseudo-notions of knowledge, truth, progress – and being able to say what is in someone else's best interests. Those 'best interests', for women with learning disabilities, have historically included being sterilized or subjected to long-acting contraceptives without explanation or choice (see also McCarthy 1994). But they can learn to name and resist the stereotypical roles into which they, like all women, have been directed to service men's needs. The group members who refused to be called out of the room to make cups of tea were resisting the same assumptions as the workers in the groups for child witnesses of woman abuse, in Loosley and Mullender's chapter, who decided that the male worker would put out the snack. Crucially, though – and this helps us to avoid essentialism and the dichotomizing of gender roles and experience – there were also women in the account by the Members of Women First who had been in charge and had operated 'bad power', perhaps more so than the men they describe as doing all the talking, butting in and putting women down because they had more authority. Above this, again, though, is a layer of analysis at which the group saw that disability services have been fundamentally designed by white non-disabled men for white disabled men. Foucauldian contributions to our understanding of power (Chambon *et al.* 1999), and longer-standing ideas from Lukes (1974), mean that power must be seen as complex and often hidden from view, not in a newly over-simplified 'bottom–up' version, to replace an earlier 'top–down' model. There are many dimensions, and resistance must make sense of all of them if it is to have any effect.

Again, the experience in men's groups is somewhat different. Blacklock, Williams and Pease all write about men being challenged, or challenging themselves, to exert less agency over others and working in alliance with women to rectify a series of imbalances, among which sex-role stereotyping traditionally gives women a lesser deal.

Deconstructing discourses

It is fascinating to be given a window onto the deconstructing and reconstructing of language that went on in the group for women with and without learning disabilities described by the Members of Women First. Not only did the women write down and physically destroy the linguistic labels that had been attached to them, but they learned together in the group that being constructively confronted within a shared groupwork process is not a personal 'put down' but is part of being valued and treated as an equal, not patted on the head and patronized as not knowing any better. Discourses that were deconstructed and questioned also included the ideas that disabled people are supposed to be grateful for services, however inappropriate and unwanted, and that women, especially disabled women, are meant to be compliant and not to get angry. This connects into Schiller's relational model (Chapter 2), where women are seen as often needing to build considerable trust before they can fruitfully engage in conflict of ideas in the group. Is this essentialist, or does it merely illustrate that dominant discourses about disability and about women have an effect in the lives of many, many individuals in interconnected, if not identical, ways? The Members of Women's First each told her story, and they were proud to be themselves, but found shared strengths within this. They also wanted to own their discourse in the group, not to have it taken away and used by others as the basis of their careers, books and fashionable practice ideas. Members of the group have owned, written and agreed the content of their own chapter in the present volume, which stands as testimony to their achievements.

The groupworker's skills, not only in helping people tell their stories but in drawing out commonalities and differences between them, is part of deconstructing and reconstructing accounts. There is a good example in Chapter 12, by Gray and Healy, where 'caring for' becomes 'caring about', which need not mean personally doing everything for the relative on every occasion, but may mean ensuring that it is done, and done to a high standard while also retaining a life for oneself. The word 'ought' is a prime candidate for deconstruction in everyone's life, and we can all feel better if we stop saying it. There is political as well as personal content in the constructions of language, of course, as Dooley and Cox show in relation to caring and ageing and as Pollio and Edmond do in the field of homelessness. In the UK, recently, we have been told that the number of rough sleepers on the streets is falling, but we know that those single people and families who are put into hostels or bed and breakfast accommodation are no longer counted as 'homeless', even though they have no settled place to live and nowhere to call their own. Language can be used to obscure as much as to clarify.

Blacklock talks about deconstructing abusive men's beliefs around their 'entitlement' to be selfish, jealous and controlling within the relationship with their partners. This is reliant on demonstrating that gender-based expectations are historically and contextually situated. They can change in a society over time and, also, within a relationship. They are not determined by biology or destiny. As we saw above, a female worker within the group can deconstruct an incident by getting the man to think about the impact his behaviour had on his partner, and often the children, not just on himself, which would be his habitual orientation. It is about reconstructing the version of masculinity by which a man lives his life, an idea more fully developed by Pease in his chapter on profeminist groups in which he shows that it is possible to challenge gender inequality both through coming together in groups and in the way we live. Interestingly, this is as much about the personal being political as is the history of feminist and social action groups, outlined by Cohen in Chapter 3. Pease puts the personal very firmly in political context by arguing that it is not enough to become a 'new man'; that man needs to live within new laws, new forms of social organization, and so on, before women can be sure of a fairer deal.

What place for groups?

In the account by the Members of Women First, it is quite clear that, while difference and diversity are firmly acknowledged and celebrated, there are enough commonalities between women, within and beyond the group, to build something together. The group members found tremendous strength and renewal in this recognition. While individuals were able to tell their stories, and be proud of who they are as individuals, they also enjoyed coming together and gained an immeasurable amount of benefit from doing so.

Groups can, of course, do harm as well as good because they are fertile and powerful contexts for influence and change. Both Pease and Blacklock refer to the risks of collusive alliances against women in all-male groups which can become self-indulgent (feeling oppressed as men, getting stuck at the guilt-tripping phase, undertaking ritualistic male bonding) if they do not constantly remind themselves (or receive reminders from groupworkers) about sexism and men's responsibility for it, often in the form of abuse and violence. Pease worries about losing engagement with accountability to women's groups and organizations, and there is a similar concern in Blacklock's idea of alliance with women workers and responsibility to female partners. So the parameters of men's groups must be clear and agreed.

Where the personal and the political are both in play, social action groups come to the fore, as Cohen highlights in Chapter 3. This is clearly demonstrated by Pollio and Edmond, also, who take a social issue with one of the profoundest possible personal effects, being without a home, and immediately show its political aspects, not only in the provision of affordable housing but in closely connected matters such as the right to vote. Group goals clearly need to be social as well as individual. Dooley and Cox similarly show the range of individual, interpersonal and cultural–social goals that can be pursued in groups. For example, they demonstrate care giving and care receiving to be public as well as private issues, and housing, health and social care policies all as matters of particular relevance to older women.

Is there, then, only one model or method available when gender is of major concern in the group, and what does the book as a whole tell us about process issues in contemporary gendered groups?

Gender and group process

In Chapter 1 and in Pease's chapter, we can see that all models and methods can be used with women and all with men. It is not sex (or gender) that determines the choice or its appropriateness. However, Cohen shows, as also do Pollio and Edmond, that some models and methods are better at helping women to question sex role and other stereotypes than others – particularly social action groups in which recruitment, structure, content and facilitation are more open, and where the expertise, strengths and goals of group members can be recognized. We also know that work with perpetrators of violence against women is best pursued in groups that combine re-educational content with space for discussion and reflective re-learning.

Overall, though, there is great variation in this volume in terms of group programme and group structure, and in the models, methods and techniques used. This was our intention, since we wanted to see how widely gender had a relevance in groupwork, not to be prescriptive about the locations or ways in which it should be raised. The conclusion we have reached is that there is an argument for regarding gender as relevant in *every* groupwork context, clearly more so in some than in others – for example where the purpose of the group is to confront gendered crime such as the abuse of women in the home or to raise women's own awareness. But in any setting where men or women, or both, facilitate groups of men or women or both – that is, in all groups – gender issues will arise and the workers need to be sufficiently alert and skilled to deal with them.

Theoretical underpinnings

The theoretical or philosophical basis underpinning the groups in this volume also varies but, more often than not, feminist or profeminist ideas are openly acknowledged, for example by Loosley, Pease, Pollio and Edmond, and Dooley and Cox, though 'feminist groupwork' does not appear to survive in the flourishing forms it took in the 1980s and early 1990s (Butler and Wintram 1991). The heritage is clearly very strong, however, and there is every reason still to value and learn from it. The Members of Women First additionally took a stance grounded in the social model of disability, while Dooley and Cox adopt the perspective of critical gerontology. These are further fruitful examples of diversity and of overlaps and interactions at work since, for disabled women and older women, two broad sets of ideas are required adequately to theorize their situation. While postmodernists might question such 'meta-narratives', or grand explanatory theories, denying their importance – provided they are taken in their more complex form, allowing for diversity within each – would seem to be to risk falling into the trap of a fragmentation that denies the advances of these critical theories over earlier individualistic and authoritarian alternatives and that side-steps the larger-scale questions of social justice (Harris 2001).

Group development

Schiller, in her chapter, shows how previous ideas on group development did not fit with a feminist theoretical base so that a new view of the stages in groups needed to be taken. She pushed at the boundaries of the 'one size fits all' model of stages in groups by looking at the woman's experience. This is the one area of group process that has been truly altered by gendered thinking and widely adopted in its new form, as an alternative to the traditional versions that preceded it. Her insights provide the nearest thing we currently have to a standardized model for working with women.

In fact, though, a number of the contributors to this volume, including Gray and Healy, and Pease, take the relational model beyond its original location of all-female groups by arguing that it may also work better in mixed groups and in profeminist all-male groups, respectively. Like Schiller, they see theoretical, practical and ethical questions in what we understand to be happening in a group and how we intervene at any particular point. Reflexivity is crucial. We need to be aware of our own gender identity and gender politics in deciding when to speak, when to redirect the discussion, and when to remain silent. Our own multiple subjectivities will inform these choices, as much as they affect the participation of group members.

Group leadership

Both Blacklock and Loosley discuss the debates around the sex of groupworkers where gender is high on the agenda in a group. Loosley reminds us that women and girls who have been sexually abused may not feel comfortable with a male groupworker and that it is more usual to have women undertaking this work. Blacklock talks about debates over whether to have two male workers or a man and a woman, Loosley whether to have all-women worker teams or a woman and a man. There have also been rare instances of two women co-working perpetrators' groups. This happened by accident in one programme I visited when a male worker was unavailable, but the woman worker who, instead, went into the group with a female colleague afterwards chose always to work in that configuration, finding it infinitely more supportive and not reliant on planning and debriefing to ensure that she was never isolated in the group. A successful 'graduate' of one of her groups remarked that, if he could survive the level of challenging in that group, becoming non-violent at home was easy in comparison. Other men might find this too much and experience it as more difficult to change without a worker they can identify with in the group; but, given the extent to which male groupworkers in perpetrators' groups have to guard against collusion with group members, this might be seen as worth the risk, at least as one co-working option. Perhaps long-term evaluations (Mullender and Burton 2001) could compare the efficacy of these various gender permutations. (And it is interesting that anti-racist work is normally undertaken by all-black teams, not black and white, so why not anti-sexist work by women?)

Blacklock gives a helpfully detailed insight into the roles that male and female workers respectively play in raising group participants' awareness of gender issues. Loosley, too, talks about ensuring that a male and female do not model stereotypical gender roles in front of impressionable children who have already seen these reinforced through violence in the home. Rather, the group can be a site of new learning about what men and women can do, and how they can co-work together effectively and sensitively. Loosley talks about the male groupworker putting out the snack, the female groupworker introducing at least half the exercises, and the two of them modelling a respectful and egalitarian relationship within which it is possible to disagree safely without being abusive. Similarly, Blacklock talks about sharing out the presentational tasks in the group by thinking through what kind of impact each worker would have in the group and how this choice can be used to maximize learning. Within this, male practitioners working with perpetrators of woman abuse can draw far more easily on their own experiences than can women, provided they are critically reflexive about these. For a female worker who shares anything negative or intimate about herself, there is the risk of voyeurism or condemnation. She, on the other hand, is more able to put forward female perspectives, including helping the men to think how their partners might react. How the male and the female groupworker interact is constantly on view in a group and requires enormous care in planning, skilled co-working and debriefing. In particular, the male worker needs to ensure that his female co-worker is never left isolated to deal with sexism – he should always step in to back her up – while the female group leader keeps a sharp look-out for any hint of collusion on the part of the male. Working at this level of intensity is only possible if each practitioner has resolved his or her own gender issues and they have also developed an equal and respectful working relationship between them. No wonder that workers in this field are shocked when agencies throw undertrained volunteers or inexperienced workers into this kind of work without adequate preparation or support (Respect 2000).

Williams's chapter on African American men in perpetrators' groups also raises controversial issues about gender and leadership skills. It is part of the received wisdom in this area of work that men must be kept to a tight focus on their violence against women and their own responsibility for it. Anything else is seen as a potential diversion from the work in hand. Thus, issues around substance misuse, families of origin, the woman's behaviour towards the man, or anything else in his current context, are usually seen as playing into his tactics of minimization and denial – allowing him to project blame onto anything and everything other than his own choice of how to think and act in a situation where he becomes abusive and violent (Mullender 1996). It is true that some of these other issues are acknowledged as needing work in their own right, for example a serious alcohol problem, but this would typically happen before, or in parallel to, membership of a perpetrators' group. Williams's argument, that the interaction between abusing women and being racially abused by a predominantly white society is a link worth making in the group, is a contentious one. It makes sense in the context of the discussion of interacting diversity throughout this book, but it is also dangerous. As he stresses, it can only be safely used in the hands of a skilled groupworker who knows how to bring the discussion back, every time, to the man's own behaviour towards his partner and to his sole responsibility for that. Done well, this could be more challenging rather than less. The man may see that his experiences as a black person are understood and addressed in the group, and yet he is *still* held to account for what he has done. He is permitted no excuse, no easy way out. This brings us back to the renewed call for a valuing of skilled and sensitive groupwork and groupworkers, to which we will return below.

Not all groupworkers practise in contexts where they have to exercise such control over process. McLeod talks about a group in which the facilitator held things together over time, since women attending did not always feel terribly well, but the members could, and did, take over the agenda when they chose. The groupworker in Gray and Healy's 'Group B' was used to a similarly low-key style and admits that she was not prepared for the difference it would make to the group dynamics when a man joined the carers' (caregivers') group. Because she was thrown by this, she omitted to promote member–member relationships and identification and to limit confrontation in the initial stages. As a result, difference rather than commonality came to the fore early on. This is a reminder of how rapidly the groupworker has to make judgements about how much to intervene and in what ways, as well as about the level of preparation that has to go into doing this well. Gendering our thinking (albeit in a more sophisticated way than previously, to allow for diversity and reframed thinking about power) is a crucial part of this. The worker's level of awareness and skills in pacing, responding, guiding, supporting and challenging are all constantly on show in a group and need to take account of gender-related issues in both content and process.

Group members

Loosley provides lively and valuable examples of helping girls to be powerful in the group and showing boys that they can learn from girls. She also talks about not having a lone male or female member, particularly in a group where gender considerations are so much to the fore. Interestingly, Blacklock talks about the formalized responsibility that perpetrator groups take towards the female partners of men in the group. Though they are not members of the programme, these women can be helped or harmed by the groupwork undertaken and their safety is accepted as top priority, taking precedence over the man's right to confidentiality in the group, for example. For a similar reason, because it is the interests of women, not of men, which take priority, the male groupworker must be allied with the woman or women in the room (and beyond it: the men's partners, and women more generally), and not with the men. There is an ever-present risk of collusion with the denial and minimization of the abuse the men in the group have perpetrated, its seriousness and unacceptability. The members, in turn, see challenges by the female worker as a put-down of all men by all women. It is important, argues Blacklock, to remain respectful towards them as people, even while challenging their attitudes and behaviour. Otherwise it is not possible for them to move forward.

Philip, in Gray and Healy's 'Group B', took centre stage, as the only man in the group, and 'quickly became the most vocal' (p. 147) which drove the women present into tending to be silent or to defer to him. The men who met jointly with the Members of Women First in other contexts, outside the group, tended to butt in and put the women down. It is not essentialist to recognize these as sex-role stereotypes because, although they do occur, they are not fixed and unchanging and because some women do these things to some men. Also, there is research evidence that women initiate interaction less and are talked to less in mixed groups than in all-female groups (see Yancey Martin and Shanahan 1983 for a summary). In Gray and Healy's Group B, the worker could have intervened in ways that helped the women become more confident and assertive, while encouraging Philip to keep his challenges until the point was reached in the group where others were ready to help him reframe them. While sex roles are not determined – Philip, as a man giving care, is a good example of this – sexist assumptions can be internalized by both men and women, and this requires that the groupworker should gender his or her intervention in the group. As Gray and Healy illustrate, this is about bringing gender to the surface and identifying gendered values and inequities so as to help all group members to examine and rethink them. The Members of Women First, in their chapter, also illustrate how internalized oppression can make women in professional and caring (caregiving) roles exercise 'bad power' in imposing services or care that are not what people really want.

A way forward for groupwork and collective action for change

One practice context in which groupwork particularly survives is domestic violence where there are groups for women, for children and for male perpetrators throughout the English-speaking world. The publication of manuals for this work has led some to assume (and we and our contributors have shared this fear; see Blacklock, for example) that groupwork skills have been diluted and that all that was left was a somewhat mechanistic approach to working through a set content from week to week – groupwork as a context but not as an instrument of change (Ward 1998). It is clear, however, from the chapters by Blacklock, Loosley and Mullender, and Williams that groupwork skills and process are alive and well in the best of these groups. We also have evidence from research (alluded to by Blacklock) that good old traditional groupwork skills do make a difference to outcome, provided they are used within a gendered perspective. We could even claim that they probably save lives. The men in Gondolf's comparative study (1998) of perpetrators' programmes were more likely to show attitude change if they had learnt to avoid violence through discussion or respect for women and their point of view. Where men said they had avoided further violent incidents by having learnt to talk things through, this was statistically linked with the one-third of women who reported 'a great extent of change' in their partners. Those women who reported 'some extent' or 'a great extent' of change were less likely to have been re-assaulted and more likely to be still with their partners. Teaching men to talk things through with their partners requires a high level of groupwork skill. This is supported by Dobash et al. (2000), based on what perpetrators said had had most effect on them in two programmes evaluated in Scotland, which revealed that the nature of the discussion in the group had been as, or more, influential than the programme content:

> Group work it seems is very important in providing a context in which violence can be discussed with others who have had similar experiences and with group leaders who focus clearly on the offending behaviour and provide new ways of seeing and understanding violence.
>
> (Dobash et al. 2000, p. ix)

In the chapters by Blacklock and by Loosley and Mullender, we see groupworkers making sensitive and subtle judgements about every word group members speak and every response they themselves make in reply. The way that child witnesses of woman abuse are helped to reconsider questions of gender-related power and control in the wider society and in their own lives, even through the simplest of games or exchanges in discussion, is a textbook example of how anti-sexist awareness can inform our practice in valuable and effective ways. Frighteningly, there are groups out there that tackle the kinds of issues described by Blacklock, Loosley and Mullender, and Williams without gendering their content. Loosley, for example, talks about a group programme that borrowed from her own but diluted its topic into 'family violence' rather than 'woman abuse'. Perhaps this book will help to demonstrate why that can be dangerous as well as wasteful of some of the best developed skills and most critical thinking anywhere in social work.

Beyond domestic violence, have women's and men's groups receded into a golden era? Certainly, several of the contributions to this edited collection have a foot in the past, notably the overview chapters by Cohen and Pease, the examples used by Lewis and Gutiérrez, and even the chapter by the Members of Women First. Does this mean that the flowering of women's groups is over? Far from it, it would seem. The illustrations developed by McLeod, Pollio and Edmond, and Dooley and Cox are all contemporary and show no less concern with women meeting together to share concerns, albeit with considerable diversity within the commonalities they share (often beyond gender alone). And there is important gender content in the mixed groups outlined by DeLois, Gray and Healy, and Loosley and Mullender, as also in the contemporary men's group examples from Pease, Williams and Blacklock. Several contributing authors are currently in practice and are writing about tensions and dilemmas they and their colleagues face on a daily basis, notably Blacklock, Loosley and DeLois. Although it was a little harder for us to find encouraging group examples of gender-based practice than it might have been ten years ago, this book stands as a clear justification for groupworkers to exercise their own social agency and bottom–up resistance in the face of managerialism, backlash and the diluting of the social work knowledge base to carry on 'thinking group' and thinking gender in groups.

It is time to revisit the undoubted strengths of feminist groupwork – the coming together as women, the awareness raising and challenging of control and domination that we saw in Cohen's chapter on feminist and women's social action groups, the sharing of commonality combined with celebration of difference and diversity – but in a new version that does not assume one justice or one truth for all women. There are arguments for seeing women's health and welfare as grounded in universal, transcultural and objective human need (Doyal and Gough 1991) and women's safety as a human rights issue (Bunch and Carrillo 1992), which makes it perfectly possible to pursue shared aims for social change. We can recognize diverse women's voices as emerging more clearly from new social movements (Charles 2000) than from older redistributive perspectives (Fisher and Kling 1994). Mullaly suggests that we can take our *ends* from the undeniable fact that many of the world's women are still oppressed, and our *means* from their ability to resist and challenge at local and global levels (Mullaly 2001). Women's collective expression, first of their despair and confusion and then of their anger (Members of Women First, Chapter 10, this volume; Leonard 1997; Mullaly 2001), can be an effective starting point for raising their voices collectively through groups. And there are encouraging signs that postmodernist ideas on power, poststructuralist approaches to alternative discourses, and feminist practice can be combined in groups that offer a new way forward. One exciting example of this is the use of narrative therapy with adult survivors of childhood sexual abuse where women resist a sense of powerlessness through telling their stories, reflecting on their feelings, and rewriting their relationships (Linnell and Cora 1993). The aim is for women to 'get in touch with a sense of themselves as experts' (p. 110) so that, without taking responsibility for another's sexual violence against them, they can take charge of their own lives. Clearly, then, there are feminist models for twenty-first century groups.

Conclusion

This book has rediscovered the true strengths of a gendered approach to social groupwork, particularly in the skills of groupworkers. They have an enormous amount to offer in practice, educational and organizational settings, where their understanding of complex interactional dynamics and their facilitation and leadership skills can bring out the best in a wide diversity of people and can, most importantly, harness energies for change.

As long as we think in terms of the multiple strengths that are present in the overlapping and interacting diversities within any group, and not in essentialist or dichotomized categories, and provided we do not ground our approach in an assumption that there are universal answers to any human problems, then there is no reason why coming together in groups should not make men more able to rethink their social positioning and women to feel stronger. If we consider, for example, the collective lifetimes of experience and wisdom that are combined in a group of older women, this represents a tremendous resource for problem solving, interpersonal support and shared action. To neglect this is to neglect the best of human agency for change.

References

Bunch, C. and Carrillo, R. (1992) *Gender Violence: A Development and Human Rights Issue*, Dublin: Attic Press.

Butler, S. and Wintram, C. (1991) *Feminist Groupwork*, London: Sage.

Chambon, A.S., Irving, A. and Epstein, L. (eds) (1999) *Reading Foucault for Social Work*, New York: Columbia University Press.

Charles, N. (2000) *Feminism, the State and Social Policy*, Basingstoke: Macmillan.

Dobash, R.E., Dobash R.P., Cavanagh, K. and Lewis, R. (2000) *Changing Violent Men*, London: Sage.

Doyal, L. and Gough, I. (1991) *A Theory of Human Need*, Basingstoke: Macmillan Education.

Fisher, R. and Kling, J. (1994) 'Community organization and new social movement theory', *Journal of Progressive Human Services*, 5, 2: 5–24.

Gondolf, E. (1998) 'Multi-site evaluation of batter intervention systems: how batterer programme participants avoid reassault', Paper presented at the Sixth International Conference on Family Violence, Durham, NH, 12 January 1988, available online at: www.iup.edu/matti/publication.

Harris, P. (2001) 'Towards a critical post-structuralism', *Social Work Education*, 20, 3: 335–50.

Leonard, P. (1997) *Postmodern Welfare: Reconstructing an Emancipatory Project*, London: Sage.

Linnell, S. and Cora, D. (1993) *Discoveries: A Group Resource Guide for Women Who Have Been Sexually Abused in Childhood*, Haberfield, NSW, Australia: Dympna House Inc.

Lukes, S. (1974) *Power: A Radical View*, London: Macmillan.

McCarthy, M. (1994) 'Against all odds: HIV and safer sex education for women with learning difficulties', in Doyal, L., Naidoo, J and Wilton, T. (eds) *AIDS: Setting a Feminist Agenda*, London: Taylor & Francis.

Mullaly, B. (2001) 'Confronting the politics of despair: toward the reconstruction of progressive social work in a global economy and postmodern age', *Social Work Education*, 20, 3: 303–20.

Mullender, A. (1996) *Rethinking Domestic Violence: The Social Work and Probation Response*, London: Routledge.

Mullender, A. and Burton, S. (2001) 'Dealing with perpetrators', in Taylor-Browne, J. (ed.) *What Works in Reducing Domestic Violence? A Comprehensive Guide for Professionals*, London: Whiting & Birch.

Respect (2000) 'Statement of principles and minimum standards of practice', available from DVIP, PO Box 2838, London, W6 9ZE.

Ward, D. (1998) 'Groupwork', in Adams, R., Dominelli, L. and Payne, M. (eds) *Social Work: Themes, Issues and Critical Debates*, Basingstoke: Macmillan.

Yancey Martin, P. and Shanahan, K.A. (1983) 'Transcending the effects of sex composition in small groups', in Reed, B.G. and Garvin, C. (eds) *Groupwork with Women/Groupwork with Men*, New York: Haworth Press (published concurrently as *Social Work With Groups* 6, 3–4).

Index